Life201
BREATHE

YOUR PATH TO IMPROVED WELLNESS
IS ONLY A BREATH AWAY

Adiel Gorel with
eight health experts

PROGRESS PRESS
SAN RAFAEL, CALIFORNIA

Progress Press
165 North Redwood Drive, Ste #150
San Rafael, CA 94903
icgre.com
info@icgre.com

This book is for educational purposes only. It is not intended as a substitute for medical or financial advice. Please consult a qualified healthcare professional for individual health and medical advice, and please consult a qualified financial professional for financial advice. Neither Ideal Life Press nor any author shall have any responsibility for any adverse effects arising directly or indirectly as a result of the information provided in this book.

This book contains the ideas and opinions of its authors. The strategies outlined in this book may not be suitable for every individual, and are not guaranteed or warranted to produce any particular results.

No warranty is made with respect to the accuracy or completeness of the information contained herein, and the authors, the publisher (Progress Press), Life201, Inc., Allusa Investments, Inc., and International Capital Group (ICG) specifically disclaim any responsibility for any liability, loss or risk, personal or otherwise, which is incurred as a consequence, directly or indirectly, of the use and application of any of the contents of this book.

Throughout this book, trademark names are used. Rather than put a trademark symbol after every occurrence of a trademark name, we use names in an editorial fashion only, and to the benefit of the trademark owner, with no intention of infringement of the trademark.

Life201 BREATHE: Your path to improved wellness is only a breath away / Adiel Gorel. — 1st edition.
ISBN 978-1-7324494-5-9 paperback edition
Library of Congress Control Number: 2022921279

ACKNOWLEDGMENTS

It has been such a gratifying experience to create this guide for a richer and fuller life, working with the expert partners who generously shared their knowledge in the chapters of this book.

Naturally, it took a village to accomplish this task!

Thanks to the incredible experts who joined me in making this useful resource on breathing for everyone:

Thanks to Dr. Nathan Bryan for his illuminating information on nitric oxide production in our bodies.

Thanks to Patrick McKeown for explaining about CO_2, breath holds, the BOLT score, and nose breathing.

Thanks to Andi and Jonathan Goldman for teaching us about the benefits and possibilities of humming.

Thanks to Beth Greer for alerting us to the many toxins we could inhale in our own homes, and showing us how to minimize exposure to toxins.

Thanks to Anat Baniel who is teaching us to change our brain via gentle movement, improving our physical and overall well-being, and creating space for better breathing.

Thanks to Dr. Erlene Chiang for teaching us about breathing and Qi, and how to live and breathe in harmony with nature's cycles.

Thanks to Jacob McGill for teaching us how to use back breathing, breathing in overall pain management, and specific breathing exercises.

Thanks to James Nestor who, in his interview with me, shared about the study at Stanford on nose breathing, talked about chewing, and the many insights his travels revealed. Although he does not have a chapter in this book, his interview is part of the Life 201 Breathing Summit, and it is fascinating.

Thanks to Dr. John Beaulieu, who shows us how we can regulate our nervous system with simple sound frequencies via tuning forks or other devices. He also talks about humming, nitric oxide, and certain breath techniques, tying everything we discuss together.

Many thanks to the team at my company, in the U.S. and abroad, for their constant support of our investors and for making the operation run smoothly, enabling me to have the time to create this book as well as other helpful content. Special thanks to Ciarra Herrell, Kristi Sessi, Lauralee Butler Reinke, and Carmit Sharaby.

Thanks to the talented and amazing team of Heightener, in particular Camper Bull, Canon Wing, Lorraine Evans, Aly Castle, and Ilya Farahmand. The Heightener team is the backbone of the summit, our podcast, and our outreach into the outside world. They are tireless and very effective.

Thanks to Chad Lefevre, who creates the structure around our podcast interviews, reaches out to the speakers, and makes the podcast happen, while also being present during the interviews. Chad makes the podcast and the summit feel comfortable and lets the speakers only worry about speaking and nothing else.

Thanks to Erin Saxton for reaching out to many of our interviewees and inviting them to contribute to our ever-growing universe of useful information. Erin's gravitas, coupled with her gregarious demeanor helps me connect with many fascinating experts.

Thanks to Jerry Adams, who was a driving force behind the public television show "Life 201," and has since been key to the development of our books, including this book sourced from the Life 201 Breathing Summit. Jerry leaves no stone unturned, and has a keen eye on deadlines, production, and performance.

Thanks to Paul Pavlovich for the design of the book, making some complex medical information readable and accessible.

And last but not least, special thanks to my children, Daphne and Daniel. You are a constant source of inspiration. I keep learning from you, and I appreciate that you also tolerate your often-busy dad. I love you!

CONTENTS

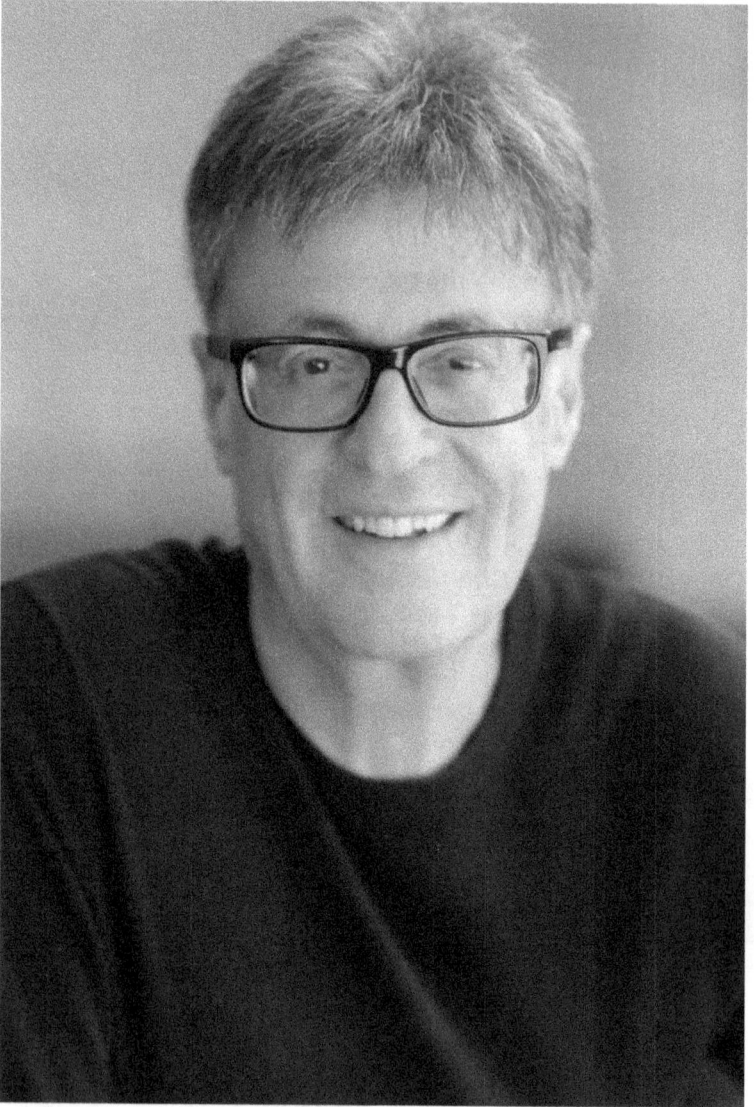

Adiel Gorel

INTRODUCTION

BETWEEN EACH PRECIOUS BREATH A NEW LIFE IS CREATED

By Adiel Gorel

Behind every breath there is a wish, to breathe in more life, health, peace, and connection to our present moment. As a life-long seeker of health and wellness, breathing is naturally one of the subjects I am interested in.

It is also my passion to inform as many people as possible about simple ways to become healthier and better quality lives. And what could be simpler than breathing?

Breathing is fundamental to our existence in the most basic way, yes, and in the most profound ways, too.

It is amazing how few of us pay any attention to this most fundamental of processes that is breathing. We breathe from the very moment of birth but many of us never give a second thought to how we do this. It is also amazing how much of a difference we could all make to our health and well-being simply by breathing correctly and consciously.

One of the ways I get the message out about this is via my podcast, where I speak to experts about their work in this field. Another way to get the message across is through this book. I have gathered some of my favorite experts on the subject of breathing and sound, to give you the most salient points on employing your breathing to improve your health.

For many years, before I explored breathing via yogic practices, I hadn't given it a second thought. I just wrote it off as one of the many automatic bodily functions. I don't need to think about it. The first time breathing became profound to me was when as a child I took a deep breath and set out to cross the length of the pool underwater as part of a game. I could feel the pressure of not breathing. I felt the exhilaration from breathing deeply after the game and the energy it gave me. For the first time, I felt I could use my breath in a way to give me more strength, or more focus, or more calm.

As a young man, I learned yoga and meditation practices, some of which included breathing. Pranayama to me was alternate-nostril breathing, as this was the one form of breathing I used before each meditation. I couldn't help but notice it always had a calming effect. No matter my mood, after a few Pranayama breaths I could feel the nervous system regulate. Still, I didn't make any concerted effort to integrate it into my daily life. I put it in a box with the yoga and never used it to help with daily stresses. Similarly, I was impressed with the deep humming of the Indian yogis, but again, their beautiful humming

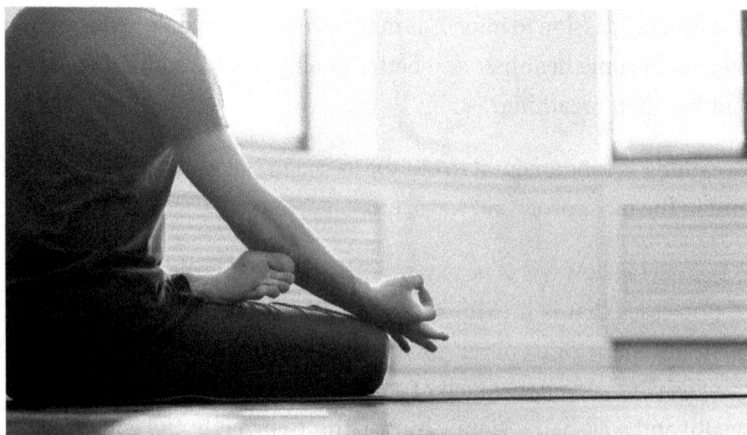

didn't seem to have a direct relevance to my own life. We can be exposed to great truths, and great healings, and yet not see them. This book is dedicated entirely to you to now see these truths in your own life.

It was in the 1980s that I was first introduced to Carl Stough, whose nickname was "Doctor Breath," by my friend and Feldenkrais teacher Anat Baniel (who also has a chapter in this book). I met Carl Stough in Manhattan, and he said I need a daily session with him for a week to get the full effect of his method. I saw him five days in a row. Each session involved exhaling while counting out loud (one, two, three, four five...), then as the exhalations grew longer (which they quickly did), singing the ABCs out loud. He was also moving my torso from side to side while I was laying on his table, to allow the diaphragm to move as freely as possible. That week was life-changing. I saw Carl Stough again several times. The walls of his office were lined with pictures of famous singers, saxophone players, and athletes, singing his praises and giving me inspiration to keep going and bring these techniques into my daily life. He had even prepared the 1968 US Olympic track team for the high-altitude Mexico Olympics. I started doing his exercises at home. In Carl Stough's opinion, the EXHALE is what's important, and the inhale is just what automatically happens after the exhale as the hunger for air reaches a certain threshold. One day I was at home, and on the TV there was an opera. The leading lady launched into a long uninterrupted song. I started at the same time as her to gauge my progress. She held on for really long, then when she was done, I continued. I managed to continue for a long time after she was done. Carl Stough's work improved the length of my exhale by that much.

I was inspired to start my podcast *The Adiel Gorel Show* after the Public Television show I had created called "Life 201." The show is still running as this book is being written. I invited experts in fields I was passionate about who inspired me, and it serves as an opportunity for me to learn more about their respective fields. The podcast allows me to interview these great experts, many of whom have dedicated their lives to a subject that could have a great beneficial effect for us. It gives me the opportunity to ask them questions, and hopefully, those Q&As are useful to a number of other people.

Continuing with the "Life 201" theme, we are holding summits on key issues. This book is part of the "Life 201 Breathing Summit." I find the experts who wrote the chapters of this book inspiring, and their material extremely useful. I try hard as I interview them to bring their knowledge "down to earth," as well as find the most useful things we can do in our daily lives with little expense or time commitment to improve our health.

Every expert who wrote a chapter in this book inspired me and changed my health in a very positive way. It is my great hope that they will inspire you. I am in deep gratitude for each and every one of these experts who took the time to share their knowledge with us in this book so that we can design our habits to serve our health throughout our lives.

Growing up, I was a part of a family of asthmatics. My father and sister being asthmatics, for a while it felt as if this was to be my fate as well. I, however, strived to not let myself be labeled in the same way, to not see myself as an asthmatic. So when my mother started me off on swimming as a young child, I stuck to it. Swimming helped me keep my budding asthma at bay. It all started with my teenage brain rejecting the labels people put on me and choosing not to accept the identity of an asthmatic.

I wasn't much of an athlete until about age 14 when the burst of testosterone related to puberty catapulted me to the realm of "not bad." Throughout my life, it was rowing, hiking, and other athletic activities that both kept me fit and the asthma well-managed.

Much of what I am today, even the motivation to put together this book, I probably owe to my grandpa. He was a health seeker himself. At the tender age of 7, I would devour my grandfather's monthly wellness magazine. It fascinated me, the idea of being big and strong and muscular like all of the people within those pages.

Having been exposed to various Pranayama techniques, and thoroughly impressed by the work I did with Carl Stough, I started developing a deeper interest in breathing.

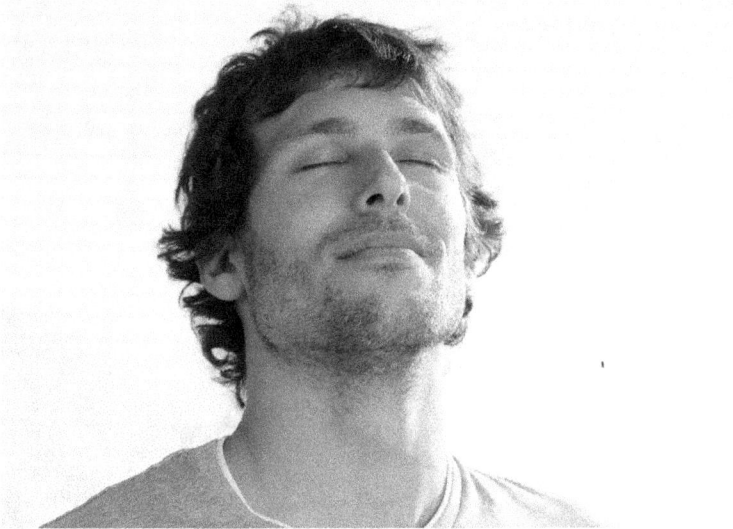

If we can breathe the way we are meant to, we can better live up to our potential. I believe that within the pages of this book you are sure to find ways to overcome your life challenges and live to your highest potential.

The message that breath can be improved is so fundamental and yet so widely overlooked. For years I have been reading up on this; becoming more and more convinced that the science is sound; the benefits to our health are clear to see.

For the last several years I have slept with my mouth taped to ensure that I breathed through my nose and not my mouth. This is based on the research about measuring bodily parameters in a sleep lab (such as the Stanford Sleep Lab), which overwhelmingly show superior results in measurements when nose breathing. It has caused a lot of hilarity for my girlfriends, but that didn't matter. I would hike up the mountain behind my house consciously breathing through the nose, which initially slowed my pace down as I accommodated to breathing that way. It didn't matter if someone called me a slowpoke. I stayed the course because I had the passion and the conviction that I was making a real difference to my health and well-being.

It is my intention for you to find in the pages of this book an increased passion for life, for finding yourself not unworthy of your vitality.

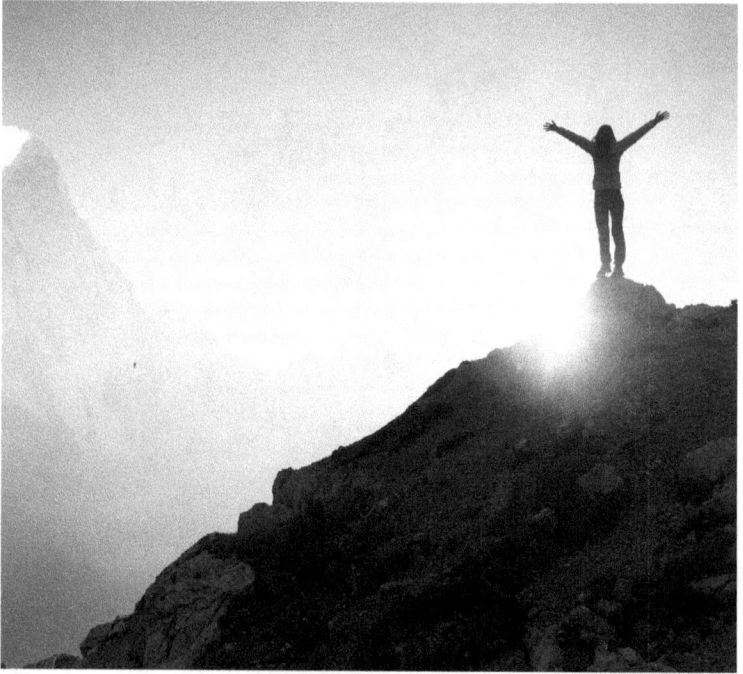

This Breathing Summit was very fulfilling for me. Being able to interview people like Erlene Chiang, Patrick McKeown, John Beaulieu, Nathan Bryan, Beth Greer, Jacob McGill, Anat Baniel, and Andi and Jonathan Goldman; to be able to pick their brains about all of the stuff I find interesting, and go as deep as I want, while also simplifying and clarifying their knowledge to make it easy and accessible to use for me, and hopefully for you.

I do not buy into the myth that we are all uniformly meant to be put out to pasture at a certain age. Just as a teenager, I didn't believe in the myth that you must resign to the label or the limits the world puts on you. I see my Qi Gong instructor who is 62. I see his flexibility and his vigor, and I feel that I would rather be like him than someone resigned to ill health due to advancing age. And breathing a certain way is a big part of practicing Qi Gong.

I have continued to find people and things and events that fascinate me, absorb me, and force me to think anew. I wish I had had the information and the insight back then that I have today. Heck, I wish I had this book back then, but I'm really grateful I'm able to bring it to you now.

I am fascinated by how breathing improves life; the way that nitric oxide plays such an important role, which became ever clearer after a trio of scientists won the Nobel Prize for their discoveries about nitric oxide and its role in cardiovascular functioning.

I started to hum more after interviewing Andi and John Goldman. Humming makes the body produce several times the amount of nitric oxide. I hum a lot, especially while driving. And, it's convenient that, despite its effectiveness, humming is free!

I invite you to dip into the labor of love of all the great experts who contributed to this book, our Life 201 book on breathing, and all the various different perspectives that all the expert writers bring to it. Maybe you don't want to devour it all at once. Maybe you want to find bits that really pertain to your lifestyle or zero in on the information that you need right now. I have endeavored to put together a comprehensive resource for you that has the potential to improve your life. I'm hoping that this work will encourage more people to breathe correctly, consciously, and healthfully.

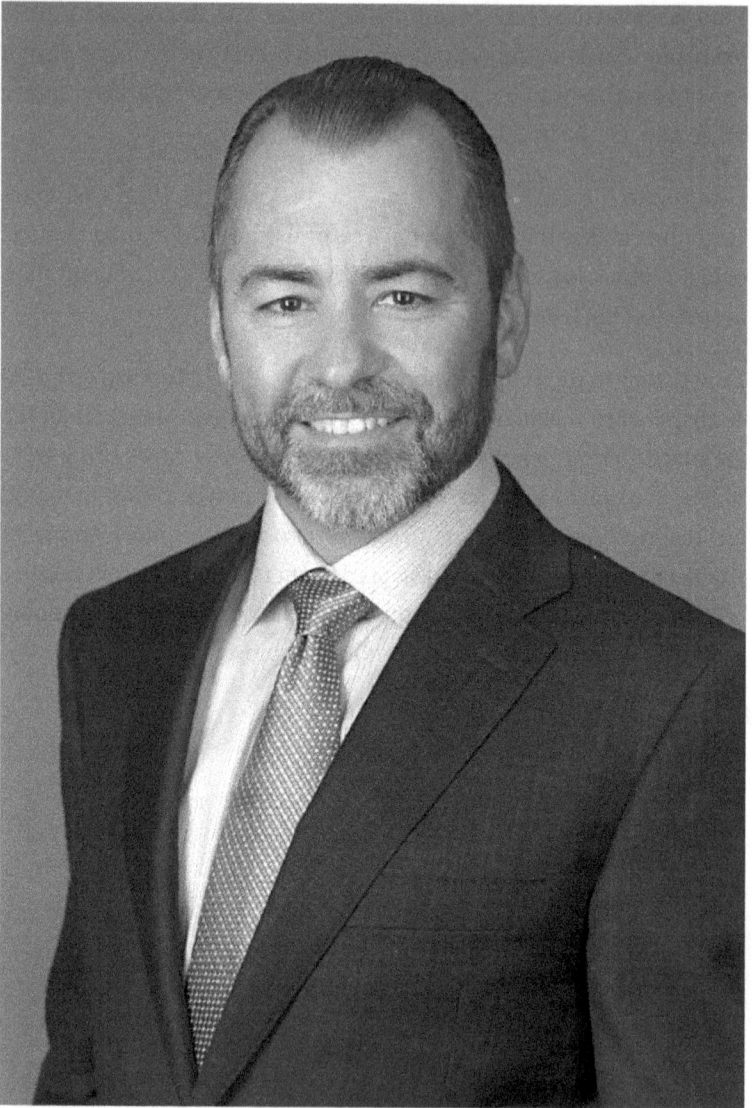

Dr. Nathan S. Bryan

CHAPTER 1

NITRIC OXIDE: *Nitric oxide **dilates blood vessels, increasing blood supply and normalizing blood pressure**. Conversely, it helps protect tissues from damage due to low blood supply. Also a neurotransmitter, nitric oxide acts in the nitrergic neurons active on smooth muscle abundant in the gastrointestinal tract and erectile tissue.*

WHAT YOU DON'T KNOW CAN KILL YOU: KNOWLEDGE IS HEALTH

By Dr. Nathan S. Bryan

Did you know that nitric oxide was discovered way back in 1772 by Joseph Priestly but that it was pretty much just dismissed as an atmospheric pollutant for two hundred years? It was much later that scientists actually discovered how vital this simple molecule – with one nitrogen and one oxygen atom – is to the human body. As late as 1998, the Nobel Prize in Physiology or Medicine was awarded to Robert F. Furchgott, Louis J. Ignarro, and Ferid Murad for their discoveries concerning "nitric oxide as a signaling molecule in the cardiovascular system."

It was about the time when I was a student at LSU School of Medicine enrolled in a Ph.D. program in Molecular and Cellular Physiology that the scientific community was waking up to the importance of nitric oxide. Even so, much remained to be understood and discovered. I had a chance to speak with Nobel Prize winner Louis J. Ignarro when he lectured at our school, and I had a lot of questions. At the time Martin Feelisch, a professor there, was also studying nitric oxide, which reeled me in to the many ways this molecule impacts our health and well-being.

We began to shine a light on the subject. What we don't know is often what kills us, and knowledge is a saving grace.

I have been studying and researching this for 22 years now, and what I have discovered points to simple but significant ways in which we can make positive changes to our health. The scientific community at large has also been delving into the many ways that nitric oxide impacts health.

How Nitric Oxide Helps With Immunity and Anti-Aging

Nitric oxide is a naturally occurring molecule in the human body. Over time and with the process of aging, production of nitric oxide naturally decreases. However, there are a lot of things we do wrong that actually hastens the process of reducing this production. We often use antacids or mouthwash, or antibiotics and other meds that inhibit production of nitric oxide. A poor diet and smoking further reduce the levels of nitric oxide in our system. The decrease in the production of nitric oxide has a direct impact on cardiovascular health – and heart disease is the number one killer of women as well as men worldwide. There is a free solution available to all, we will go into the details of which in this chapter.

This is a gas that's produced primarily in the lining of the blood vessels. It is a neurotransmitter that controls oxygen, nutrient, and blood flow delivery to every organ, tissue, and cell in the body. It's a neurotransmitter – in other words, it's how cells in the brain communicate with one another. It's also really important for our immune system. It is how our white blood cells fight off invading pathogens, whether it's viruses or bacteria, or any parasite or invading species. So when you lose the ability to generate nitric oxide, there are a lot of bad things that happen. Avoidable bad things. You develop high blood pressure, you lose regulation of blood flow, you develop sexual

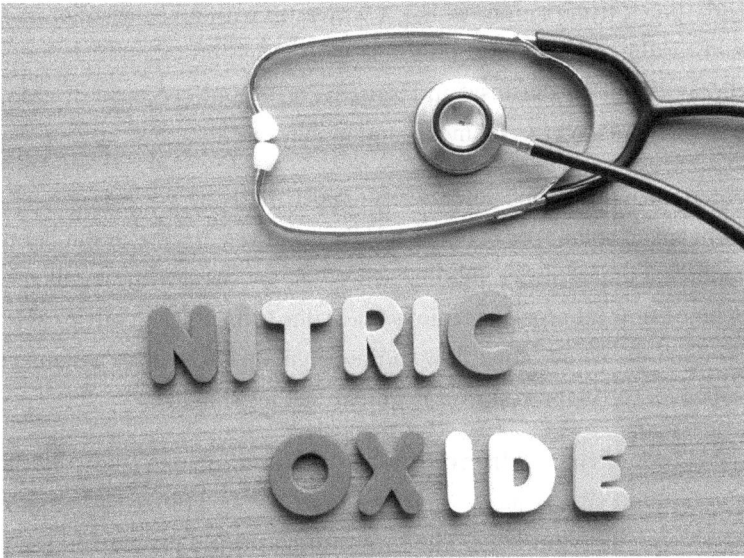

dysfunction, you become immunocompromised, you develop vascular dementia, and eventually cognitive disorders and Alzheimer's. A wide range of symptoms could actually present due to a lack of nitric oxide in the body. In fact, every single human chronic disease is associated with low blood flow and hence low nitric oxide. It's a pretty powerful molecule our bodies are perfectly set up to use as a health giver.

To put it simply, nitric oxide improves oxygen delivery and blood flow to all downstream tissue. It is needed to bind hemoglobin in red blood cells, which deliver oxygen to the periphery. So without nitric oxide, you cannot deliver oxygen to the tissues. This has proved critically important in the past two years with Coronavirus and the problem of hypoxemia – an abnormally low concentration of oxygen in the blood. You can see this in patients who, when their doctors put them on oxygen, their blood oxygen saturation does not improve until their doctors restore the functionality of nitric oxide.

Nitric oxide production is closely tied to chronic disease that we see so much of later in life. It is also tied to why kids don't have hypertension or heart disease even when they've not been eating their veggies as they should. Children have good endothelial function and are able to produce enough nitric oxide. In older adults, we see much more endothelial dysfunction, which is why even with a healthy diet and exercise the incidence of chronic disease is widely prevalent. This is the slippery slope for the onset and progression of cardiovascular disease, and even diabetes, Alzheimer's, and kidney disease.

When you reduce blood flow to every organ in the body, you're eventually going to get some type of end stage disease. Even erectile dysfunction could be a sign of nitric oxide deficiency – simply because the regulation of blood flow into specific regions is lost due to insufficient nitric oxide production. When blood flow to the pelvic region and sex organs is impeded, the blood vessels don't dilate as they should.

Similarly, if the prefrontal cortex of the brain isn't getting as much blood supply as it needs, you may not be able to remember where you left your keys. The forgetfulness could proceed to mild cognitive disorder, and then proceed onto vascular dementia and Alzheimer's disease.

Healthy Circulation Is a Key Indicator of Overall Health

When you think about it, everything ties in to the need to maintain good circulation in the body. Consider how erectile dysfunction drugs were actually first designed as heart medications since the desired outcome of both is dilation of blood vessels. There's clear evidence now that people on PDE5 inhibitors or erectile dysfunction drugs have, by some estimates, a 30% to 40% lower risk of Alzheimer's. These drugs are now approved for pulmonary hypertension as well, but they still don't get to the root of the problem, which is a lack of nitric oxide production.

How You Can Make the Health Building Molecule: Nitric Oxide

Breathing through the nose and more particularly deep breathing is an important way for the body to access this vital molecule. The enzyme found in our epithelial cells in our nasopharynx is activated when we deep breathe through our nose. Nasal breathing activates this enzyme, and so long as it's active and functional, can produce nitric oxide.

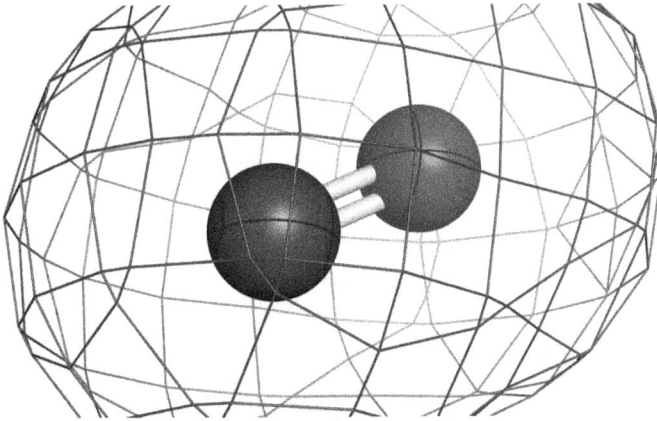

This dilates the bronchial airways and improves oxygen uptake in the lungs. So deep breathing stimulates the epithelial production of nitric oxide, and eating green leafy vegetables helps the body create nitric oxide.

You also stimulate enzymatic production through exercise, which stimulates nitric oxide production. When we exercise, whether it's weightlifting, running, or cycling, this creates sheer stress in the lining of the blood vessels. This signals the need for more oxygen and nutrients to support this increased metabolic activity of the muscle, which in turn stimulates nitric oxide production. In well-trained athletes, their ability to produce nitric oxide actually predicts their exercise capacity and their performance. This is why many athletes supplement with nitric oxide products to improve their performance.

Another important thing to keep in mind is the importance of maintaining a good, diverse oral microbiome. This means that we try not to interfere with the naturally occurring bacteria in the mouth by using mouthwash, etc. All this helps ensure that your body can produce the requisite nitric oxide every second, every minute, every hour of every day.

The reason that so many of us are nitric oxide deficient is because of endothelial dysfunction and the enzyme not working properly. This happens when we don't eat a good diet, or use a mouthwash, which disrupts that normal nitric oxide production, use antacids, and so on. And that's when people start to get in trouble.

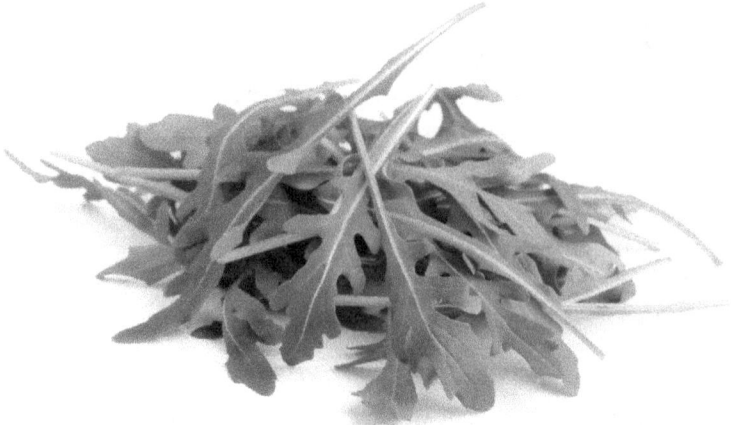

Arugula, Celery, and Cabbage... Oh My!

One of the natural and powerful ways in which the body makes nitric oxide is through this enzyme called nitric oxide synthase in our epithelial and endothelial cells. This enzyme converts L-arginine to nitric oxide. Arginine is a semi-essential amino acid, and a lot of proteins have arginine as part of their makeup. So as long as you can break down proteins (animal and plant-based) into amino acids, you're getting a source of those amino acids. Then there is a molecule called inorganic nitrate that's found primarily in dark green leafy vegetables. The darker the vegetable, the more nitrate these vegetables typically have. So, things like kale, arugula, spinach, cabbage, lettuce, and celery are rich in nitrates. And then when we consume those, the body converts that into nitrite and nitric oxide.

Is Modern Medicine Getting It Wrong?

Pharmaceutical companies claim to use restorative pharmacology, but this is something of a contradiction in terms. The idea should be to fix and correct disease using safe, effective, rationally designed therapeutics; to fix the underlying problem that causes chronic disease. However, modern medicine doesn't address the root cause of disease. Instead, it prescribes the inhibitor of a certain enzyme, and when you inhibit biochemistry, there are consequences. Those consequences are what we know as side effects. Most drugs have side effects, and in one sense, approved prescribed drugs remain a top cause of death in America.

A lot of drug commercials on TV seem to be telling us about the clinical benefits for a few seconds followed by a litany of possible side effects. The visuals, however, will cause you to believe that the drug is going to cure and restore you to good health without any of those well-documented side effects.

Think about antacids – so commonly prescribed. They may neutralize the discomfort, but they also cause lower stomach acid to be produced. This means that the body is unable to absorb zinc, iron, selenium, chromium, iodine, and the B vitamins as effectively. Studies have shown that people who have been on these acids for three to five years have about a 40% higher incidence of heart attack and stroke. So get off those antacids and let your stomach do its job. There is also a correlation between the use of mouthwash and an unsafe elevation in blood pressure.

Much of this needs to change to mitigate the negative impacts of drugs. This is why we have to change the direction in drug discovery and drug design... because the body does in fact have a powerful ability to heal itself.

How To Give the Body Back What It Needs To Heal Itself

Here's where you do your part to prevent all of those medical conditions we already spoke about, here's where you get back to your body's natural power to heal and thrive. Let's start with something as simple as diet and its impact on nitric oxide production. Some cultures traditionally have diets that support nitric oxide production. The Japanese diet, for instance, is well known for the way it promotes health and longevity.

Eating more leafy greens like kale, arugula, spinach, and celery is recommended. When you eat leafy and other greens, you're giving

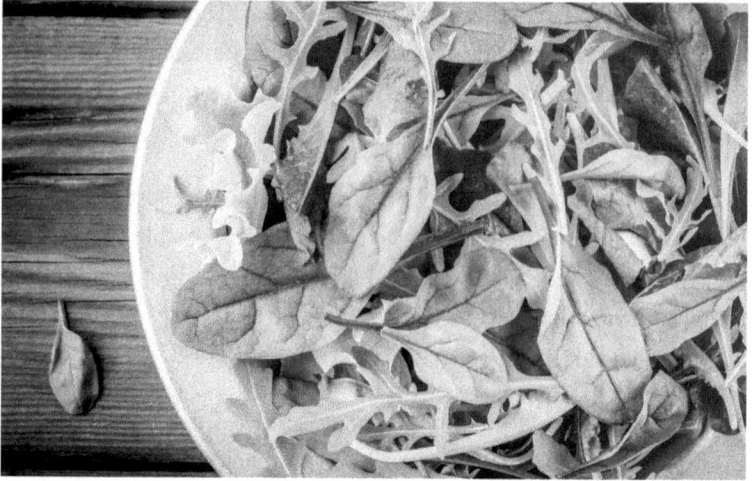

yourself a source of nitric oxide for the next six or eight hours. You also have the right oral bacteria and you can make stomach acid. That prevents postprandial oxidative stress and hence is extremely important.

It is true that some of these beneficial foods can cause bloating or discomfort when first introduced into the diet. However, the body is marvelously adaptive. It will start to accumulate the bacteria that are needed to metabolize those different foods, and the bloating will go away. The idea is to prevent dysbiosis and maintain microbial diversity of the gut. The beneficial bacteria that line the gut actually do what the body cannot do by itself. So, eating a variety of different foods helps maintain microbial diversity, ergo, gut health.

However, not all leafy greens are equal. For instance, spinach contains six times more nitrates than broccoli and almost twice that in celery. And organic isn't necessarily better here. Organic produce doesn't have herbicides or pesticides, but they may not be very beneficial because of how they tend to be deficient in many minerals and nutrients, including nitrate. The soil itself is bereft of nutrients because of our intensive farming practices.

Another important issue to touch upon is that of nitrates and nitrites, and how their presence in cured meats has been linked to cancer. There was so much alarmism around this that laws were passed to mitigate the carcinogenic impacts of cured meats. Later research, however, demonstrated that "only around 5% of nitrates in the average European diet come from processed meats, while more than 80% are from vegetables." Now we know that nitrites could actually prevent certain cancers. Further, the way that manufacturers were cutting down on the nitrites was ineffective. For instance, bacon made by adding celery powder isn't just a more expensive product, but also has higher bacteria content and a shorter shelf life. So I tell people, save your money and buy the regular cured products; simply moderate your intake.

Chewing Can Benefit Your Health Now and in Future!

We need to focus not just on what but how we eat as well. Chewing well not only helps physically break down food into more easily digestible particles but also helps maintain a healthy bacterial population in the mouth. Further, eating slowly and chewing well means you have time to signal satiety to the brain so you're less likely to overeat. Eating should be an enjoyable, social, even spiritual activity. Being distracted while eating means poor digestion and just taking away from the joy of eating.

Given that people have varied oral microbiome and stomach acid levels, different dietary patterns, and exercise regimen, they could have very diverse nitric oxide needs as well. I have been researching and working to create solutions that work for everyone, effectively and safely. Some years back, I developed an orally disintegrating nitric oxide tablet that has been successful. I currently have a number of effective nitric oxide supplements and nutritional products on the market. I also have a drug company where we're developing nitric oxide-based therapies that will be prescription medications for doctors to prescribe for specific indications.

I developed a new nitric oxide drug to help manage at-risk COVID patients with comorbidities. Our investigational new drug application was approved by the FDA in 2020. It has been very effective in keeping people out of hospital. It helps keep blood oxygen saturation from dropping. This drug is developed as an early treatment for COVID patients to keep them out of the hospital. We are also working on drugs that are going to help with dilation of blood vessels, to help with ischemic heart disease, Alzheimer's, and ischemic, non-obstructive coronary artery disease. We've even developed a topical nitric oxide serum that we brought to market as a skincare and beauty product several years ago. We also developed an innovative beet root product where we actually ferment and concentrate nitric oxide activity into the beet powder while removing the beet color, beet taste and oxalates. Significant research and development is ongoing, and we are at various stages of receiving FDA approval for the various drugs we have worked on.

I am 48 but have the vascular age of a 24 or 25-year-old. I myself use the nitric oxide tablets maybe once or twice a day depending on how I'm feeling. These tablets or lozenges give 24-hour coverage, but individual requirements may be more or less depending upon individual cases. In some cases, this may be two, or up to four or five a day for some of the more complex cases. In older people who need to take antacids, that requirement might be higher.

We have launched a product called NO Beetz that's a white beet powder. The pulp and the color are extracted and this is then fermented to effectively give users the nitric oxide benefits of the food. This obviates the need to ferment and consume large amounts of beet, which most people don't really like the taste of. So, this is a workable solution that has the concentrations of nitrate and nitrite that you need to see a physiological effect.

However, rather than try to sell my products I'm more interested in informing people about the science and the mechanism behind nitric oxide and its most effective delivery systems. For instance, a lot of athletes are using products that don't have any discernible nitrate or nitrite in them. So it really is a case of caveat emptor (buyer beware) of what they are buying.

Why Humming To Yourself Is Actually a Healthy Exercise

To increase nitric oxide production naturally, get regular exercise, change your diet to eat plenty of leafy greens, and stop using mouthwash

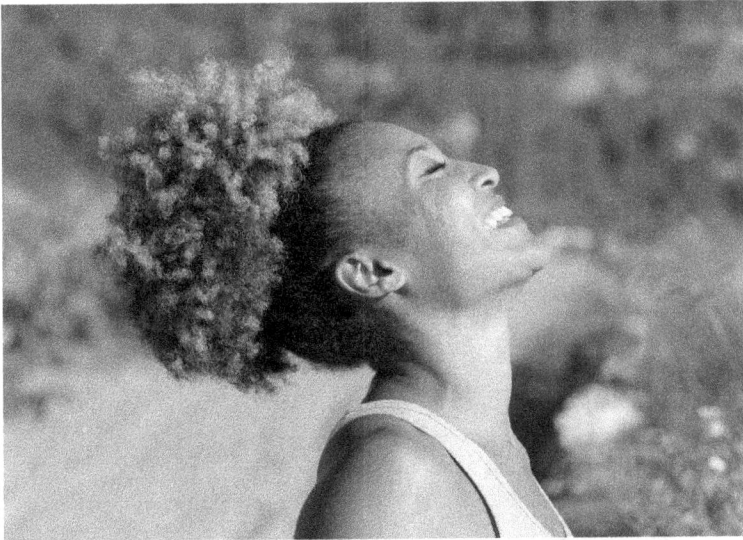

and antacids if possible. Try adding dietary supplements into the mix to help the body access and absorb nutrients more effectively. The body actually has the ability to heal itself, so long as we create an optimal internal environment to facilitate this.

Something you can do for yourself every day, simply and effectively, is breathe the right way. Deep breathing, humming, and nasal breathing are seen to make a substantive difference to nitric oxide production. While humming, for example, we can detect more nitric oxide coming out of your exhaled air, provided the enzyme is functional. Deep breathing lowers your blood pressure, which is well established, and some frequencies of songs or singing or humming can also lower blood pressure.

Breathing right is the simplest way to increase nitric oxide levels in the body.

There are over 175,000 scientific papers published on nitric oxide, and the evidence is clear that nitric oxide is a vitally important ingredient in health, healing, and destroying disease. If you would like to know more about this molecule, and the research that other experts and I have conducted into it, drnathansbryan.com is a resource that I have created for exactly this purpose.

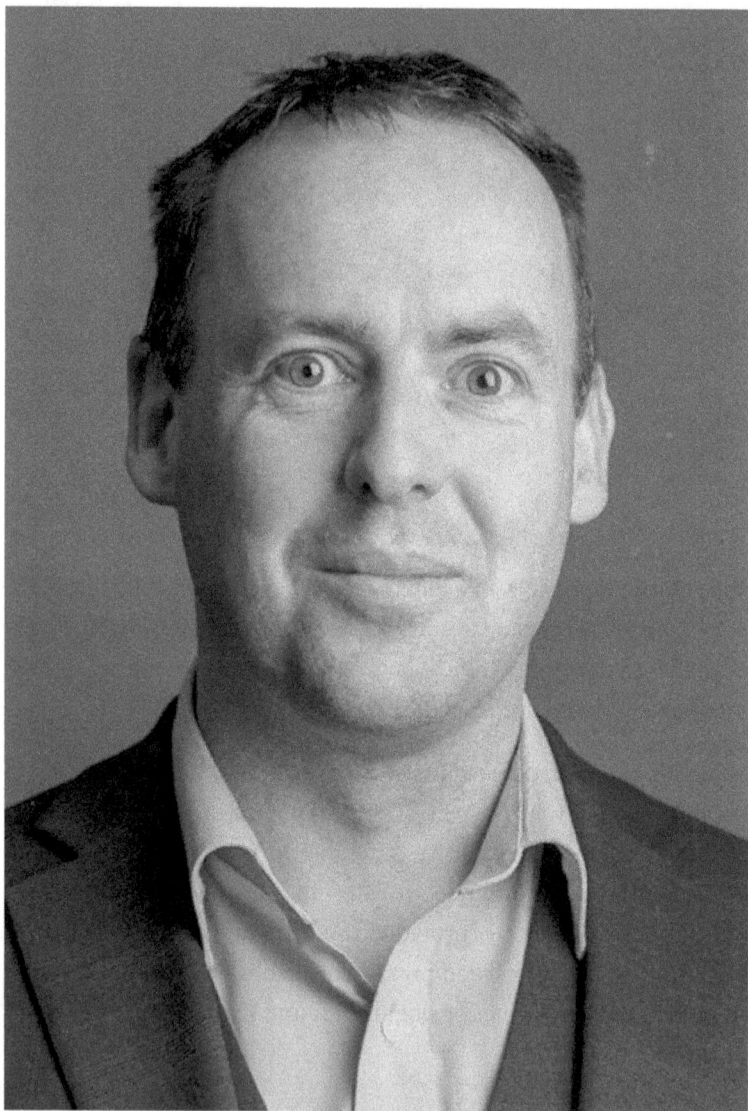

Patrick McKeown

CHAPTER 2

AIR HUNGER: *Air hunger is a hormetic or healthy stressor that, when done right, can improve breathing and result in better health overall. It is a sensation of a strong urge to breathe or a feeling of breathlessness.*

GETTING THE OXYGEN ADVANTAGE: BREATHE BETTER, FEEL BETTER

By Patrick McKeown

I was listening to the podcast *Feel Better, Live More with Dr. Rangan Chatterjee*, particularly the episode *"Life Lessons from a Brain Surgeon with Dr. Rahul Jandial."*[1] Dr. Rahul speaks about the importance of breathing being the best method for emotional regulation; about having the greatest clarity when one's breathing is under check. Breath control is his go-to rule for crisis management, says the doctor.

Now, the good doctor knows this, but why doesn't everybody else? Why doesn't the university student, nervous about going in for an exam, know it? The body recognizes faster, harder breathing as the body being under stress. Students, business people, and anyone who relies on their ability to focus is going to benefit from breath control. As Dr. Rahul says, you can train yourself to be calmer by controlling your breathing, specifically by controlling the exhalation. The body interprets fast exhalation during rest as the body under stress.

Whenever you get into a difficult or challenging situation, do your best to bring your attention inwards, onto the breath. Nobody will even know that you're doing it! The slow, relaxed, prolonged exhalation stimulates the vagus nerve, which secretes the neurotransmitter acetylcholine to help slow down the heart. The brain then interprets this slowed heart rate from the secretion of acetylcholine as the body being safe.

We think of being calm and collected, being able to come up with a good solution in a crisis as the measure of a leader. This takes training for some while it comes naturally to others. This has a lot to do with concentration – something most of us are never taught how to do. How do we concentrate? What does it take to be able to hold our attention 100% to the task at hand? Disordered breathing is not going to let us do it.

Disordered breathing while sleeping, i.e. heavy snoring, insomnia, or obstructive sleep apnea, affects a huge cohort of the population. It impacts the ability to concentrate. The physiology of dysfunctional breathing and the resultant stress response does impact concentration and much else besides. So whether it's a student, corporate worker, athlete, homemaker, or anyone, breath control is important for performance, problem-solving, decision making, and overall well-being.

Stress and Breathing – The Physiological Impacts

One of the reasons for poor concentration is that we are an always connected, "always on" culture. With all the information bombarding us, content constantly jostling for mind-space and only so many hours in the day, our attention spans are shrinking rapidly. Of course, there are people with medical conditions; there are people who have ADD and ADHD, but many have simply surrendered their attention to all the big platforms out there. The mind is racing, nothing holds the attention for long, and quality of work suffers.

Imagine going to a restaurant for a lovely meal. To really appreciate it, you have to be able to smell it, taste it, feel it, and appreciate the visual aspects of the plating, the interiors, and so on. Much of the time, however, we are so distracted that a lot of these beautiful experiences

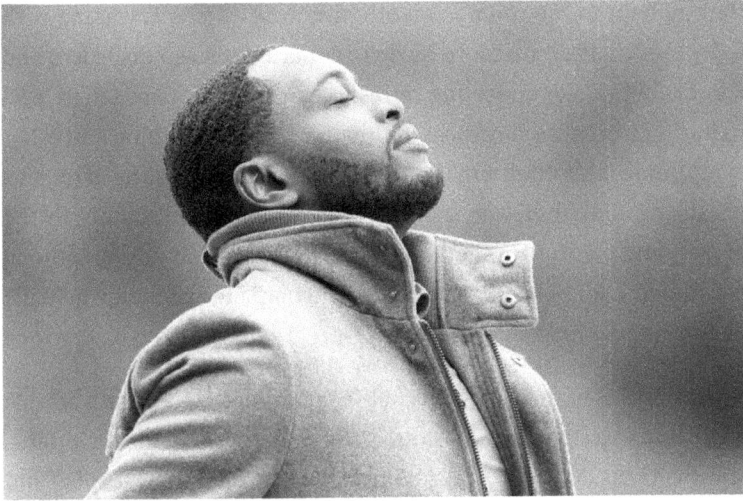

pass us by. We tend not to give our attention to the people with us because of the constant notifications, and the very presence of all the devices.

When I was fourteen, I left school. I had problems concentrating and paying attention to the teacher. My teachers told me I would be better off picking potatoes in the field than being in class.

At the time, I went off to do my own thing. The main reason I left school was that I felt like I had no energy. I had a breathing sleep disorder that kept my system in a constant state of stress.

I went back to school later, but it wasn't easy. I got my university degree and got into the corporate world but it was still difficult for me to cope. Then in 1998, I read an article about the importance of breathing – breathing through the nose and breathing right. I then changed careers and trained, or rather retrained, myself in breathing.

Breathing and the Instagram Generation

I was one of the lucky ones. There are kids, teenagers, adults...they're going through life, never reaching their full potential simply because they don't have functional breathing and are not getting good quality sleep. There is a close connection between mental health issues, poor sleep quality and breathing.[2] When it comes to sleep quality, the elephant in the room is mouth breathing. If one is waking with a dry mouth, they are more likely to experience sleep disorders and less likely to wake up feeling refreshed. Feelings of fear, stress, and irritation can cause shortness of breath or rapid breathing and other symptoms. This then creates a vicious cycle where the irregular breathing contributes to the feelings of anxiety and panic. In the anxiety and panic disorder population, a majority have dysfunctional breathing. The shallow breathing and incomplete exhalation actually feeds those feelings of anxiety.

In Maslow's Hierarchy of Needs, self-actualization is the zenith of what we as humans strive for. Maslow spoke about needing food, clothing, and shelter as our basic needs. Fortunately, most of us have this – but we don't have deep sleep. We don't have functional breathing. We don't have breath and awareness, and the ability to reach that state of bliss. We aren't able to access creativity, intuition, or ambition even though we have the ability to concentrate fully; to connect with life, see more and miss less.

And then came mobile phones, particularly the smartphones with cameras and social media. A whole generation of kids grew up with their heads literally stuck in a phone, giving all of their attention to these huge multinational platforms. It is crazy, even sinister. This should carry a health warning because of how these platforms contribute to mental health problems. Kids are dying by suicide as a result of the anxiety and pressures on them!

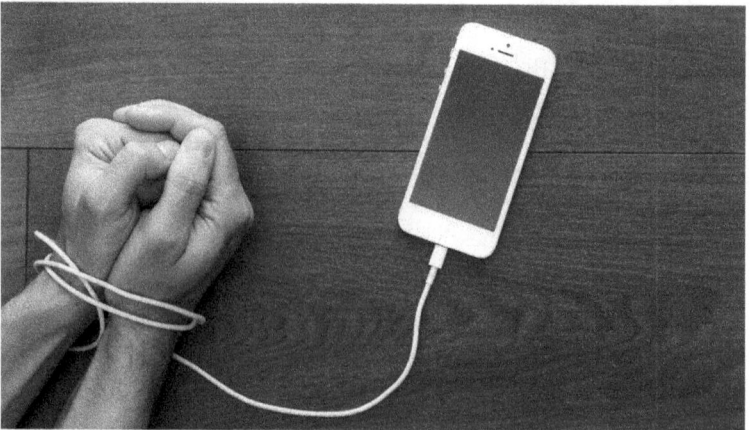

Studies have shown the detrimental impacts of social media on young people, especially Instagram, which has been seen to be the most pernicious.[3] The impacts of social networks such as YouTube, Twitter, Facebook, Snapchat and Instagram were examined. Researchers found negative impacts on sleep quality, bullying, body image and FOMO among young users. Except for YouTube, the other four networks were associated with increases in depression and anxiety as well. The phenomenon of the 'compare and despair' attitude creates dissatisfaction with one's own reality. It was found that spending more than two hours a day on social media means a higher likelihood of reporting psychological distress.

Why Haven't We Been Taught How to Breathe Properly?

Clearly breathing is fundamental, and breathing dysfunction has some very grave and far-reaching consequences. And yet, we hardly hear about it. One of the reasons for this is that we are never really taught breathing – when we are, we've been taught it wrong. There is a lot of misinformation out there. Why, for instance, does the population not know that the harder and faster you breathe, the less oxygen is delivered to the body? The idea in the general population is the opposite!

Why haven't we been taught how to breathe properly, where we can take corrective action when we are stressed, or have insomnia, and so on? Why haven't we been taught that slowing down those exhalations will calm the body; send out the message to the body that everything is OK. Slow, light and silent prolonged exhalation is a simple tool that one can discreetly apply without anyone knowing. If stress is pushing people over the edge, is there a way to resolve this? Is it possible to do this just by focusing on breathing?

These fundamental solutions have not been communicated to the general populace.

A big reason why no one seems to be talking about breathing is, it is difficult to monetize. Financial returns are slim. People are not going to make millions off telling others that mouth breathing is an emergency response, or about how it sends the body into a fight or flight response.

In my own personal experience, the medical community doesn't want to talk about this. This is despite the fact that the medical community is well aware that nose breathing filters airborne particles, regulates volume, increases oxygen uptake, plays a role in improving sleep quality and has antiviral impacts.

In 2005 I was at an asthma conference in Ireland, and I was asked not to address any questions about nasal breathing!

As an asthma sufferer for 20 years myself, I now know about the vital importance of nasal breathing and good quality sleep. And yet, no doctor ever told me about it. We as a society have overlooked the importance of nasal breathing – maybe we think it's too simple to have to learn?

How Breathing Is Linked to Various Health Parameters

Think about when you're doing something strenuous like hiking, which makes us feel breathless. If we breathe out through the nose, we start to feel air hunger, which is basically carbon dioxide being unable to leave the body quickly enough. So, when you first exercise with your mouth closed you will feel that air hunger, but over time the body will adapt to it.

Carbon dioxide is important for another reason. Hemoglobin, which is carrying oxygen, releases oxygen more readily to the tissues in the presence of carbon dioxide and lower blood pH. This is the Bohr Effect.[4] So what the nasal breathing does is, it helps oxygen delivery to the tissues and also strengthens the diaphragm by imposing resistance while breathing.

Dysfunctional breathing can cause back pain and neck pain, and adversely affects the musculoskeletal system. People with breathing dysfunction are found to have lower pain thresholds, and impaired motor control, balance, and movement. One study[5] examined the connection between breath time and dysfunctional breathing. Study participants with the Breath Hold Time (BOLT as described below) of over 25 seconds were 89% likely to have functional breathing.

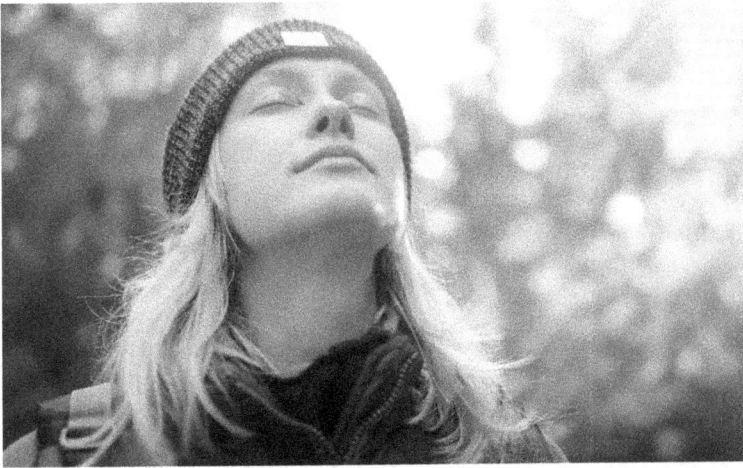

Individuals with a lower breath hold time during rest are more likely to breathe faster, breathe from the upper chest, and have increased breathlessness during physical exertion. They are more likely to breathe hard and fast during sleep because how you breathe during wakefulness will influence how you breathe during sleep. Breathing hard and fast during sleep increases turbulence in the airway, which can contribute to snoring and possibly obstructive sleep apnea.

The diaphragm is a key organ in the way it helps to stabilize the spine and also plays a role in lymphatic drainage. When we breathe with good recruitment of the diaphragm, it increases lung volume. This can have wide ranging consequences for health, managing chronic disease, athletic performance, and more. It then follows that retraining the body to breathe in the right way can help us reap tremendous benefits as well.

One of the ways to do this is to find out about the body's BOLT score. The BOLT or the Body Oxygen Level Test – is an indicator of good or suboptimal health. This test measures how long you can hold your breath comfortably. Healthy individuals with functional breathing will have a BOLT score of above 25 seconds. Low BOLT scores indicate dysfunctional breathing. We see that dysfunctional breathing can hold back even healthy people. This isn't just about getting overly breathless during physical exercise or poor athletic performance. It impacts productivity, state of mind, sleep, and resilience.

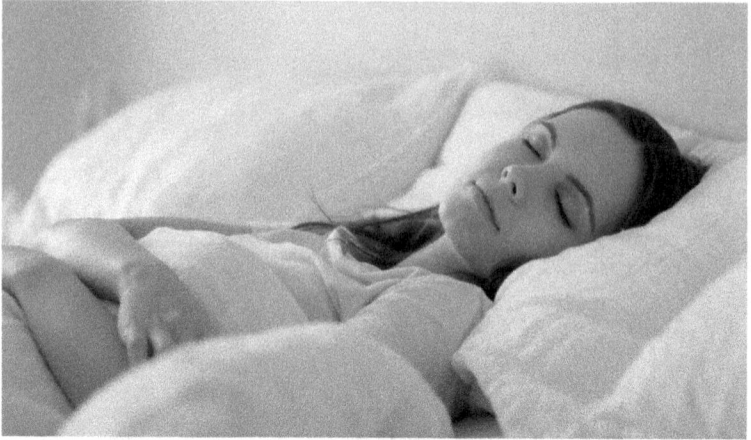

If the BOLT score is subpar, the first step would be switching to nose breathing and to have the mouth closed during sleep. Waking up with a dry mouth in the morning isn't going to be good for accessing flow states. Even just from the point of view of dental health, mouth breathers are more liable to have bad breath, gum disease, and dental cavities than nasal breathers. When you breathe in and out through your nose, your mouth is moist and saliva helps to protect your teeth and your gums. If the BOLT score is, say, 16 seconds, the person may feel well, and may even be coping quite well. But when the individual starts breathing through their nose during sleep and exercise, they will find that they are making a positive difference to their health and well-being.

I recommend that maybe the last 15 minutes or so before bed, sit down and take a very soft, gentle breath in through the nose. Follow this with a really relaxed, slow, and gentle breath out. A very soft and slow, gentle breath in through the nose, and a very relaxed and slow, gentle breath out. The breath is imperceptible. It's hardly noticeable that any air is coming into the body. As for the exhalation, aim for a totally relaxed and prolonged exhalation; imagine the diaphragm moving back to its resting position. The objective here is that you feel air hunger. There will be increased saliva production, the hands start to feel warmer, and you might start to feel a little drowsy. Now when you sleep at night, your breathing isn't going to be as hard and fast, and you're also less likely to have a stuffy nose as you sleep.

To decongest your nose, you have to hold your breath longer than 30 seconds. Pinch and hold your nose, and gently nod your head up and down or move your body and keep relaxing into the breath hold. Relax into it and keep holding your breath until you feel a moderately strong air hunger. Then let go and breathe in through your nose. Even one breath hold will open up your nose. I must mention here that it is not advisable for pregnant women or those with any serious medical conditions to create air hunger.

The Nasal Breathing Strip to the Rescue?

One of the ways to promote nasal breathing while sleeping at night is the nasal strip that works for both adults and children. This is a tape that surrounds the lips to counter the habit of mouth breathing while asleep, which happens when the mouth falls open. This is an elasticized tape that pulls the lips together without covering the mouth. It basically trains the person to breathe through the nose. It prevents mouth snoring and reduces sleep apnea while increasing Continuous Positive Airway Pressure (CPAP) compliance, and improving sleep quality and focus. It reduces symptoms of asthma, boosts oral health, and promotes relaxation and even athletic performance. You wake up just feeling better.

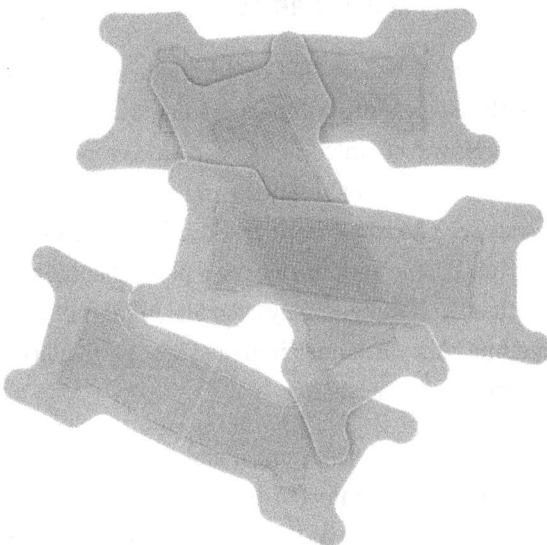

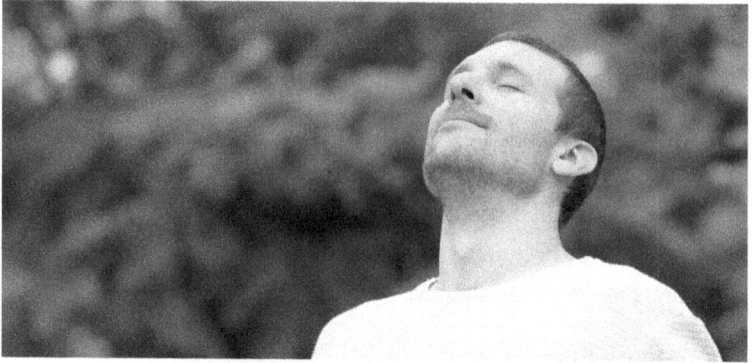

This also helps ease a stuffy nose when you do the exercise to build up your BOLT score – the nose will simply be less stuffy. Keep in mind that the nose has a normal nasal cycle where one side of the nose remains clear for about 90 minutes and then the other. We never have a completely clear nose and this is normal. However, the thing to remember is that the more we use the nose, the better it works. So if you're going to keep breathing through the mouth, this is going to contribute to nasal congestion. The thing is not to let a little nasal congestion deter you – work through it. Maybe use a nasal dilator – a little plastic device that goes into the nose to open it up and improve airflow. Some nasal dilators are adhesives that go over the nose to help the nasal passage open up.

Start Slow and Strengthen Your Breathing Over Time

Now in the West, we believe that bigger the better, more the merrier and so on – the concept of air hunger is something that has a negative connotation. However, introducing air hunger is a positive thing for all the reasons that I mentioned earlier. To be sure the feeling of breathlessness can be unpleasant and could make us uncomfortable or even fearful. People with anxiety or a panic disorder could have a strong reaction to air hunger; may even feel mildly suffocated. So this is not something that you launch into full scale, particularly if someone has a history of such disorders.

We start with a teaspoon of air hunger and we increase it by soupçons. We gently introduce discomfort in dribs and drabs; in ways that allows the body to get used to it. We do this in a controlled way to start deriving benefits from it. I don't recommend going off the deep end, I don't say we should be jumping into icy pools or suddenly stress the system. You do it gently, gradually, and you build up your capacity. When we talk about hormetic stressors (healthy stressors like cold exposure, intermittent fasting, and HIIT exercise), we go very easy because you don't know how your body will respond to them. There's no one approach and it isn't a one size fits all. When you stress your body and your mind, start with a teaspoon and go from there.

Empower Yourself by Retraining Yourself to Breathe Right

There are some powerful ways in which you can empower yourself to breathe better, be healthier, and unlock your potential. *The Oxygen Advantage*, *Asthma-Free Naturally* and *Close Your Mouth* are some of my books designed to inform and enable readers to take charge of their own well-being. *The Breathing Cure* is my book that delves into topics such as obstructive sleep apnea, children, difference between female and male breathing, epilepsy, diabetes, asthma, and panic disorder. You will find help managing and reducing the symptoms of chronic conditions. There is also a book titled *Atomic Focus*, which I wrote specially for people with ADHD. It is true that much of what I base my techniques on is scientific and technical. However, this book is designed to hold your attention: with big fonts, lots of color photos, and an easy layout.

Our workshops include live breathing classes, one-on-one training, self-study breathing courses, training for breathing in martial arts, an online sleep course, online course for anxiety, breathing techniques for females and for seniors, breathing for yogis and so on. We have about 3000 instructors across 50 countries and at oxygenadvantage. com. You'll see there's an instructor locator there. Now, we also have another website, a sister website called buteykoclinic.com.

Whether you're an athlete looking to improve performance or just someone looking to take charge of your health, stress, and well-being, you can experience phenomenal improvements just by changing how you breathe.

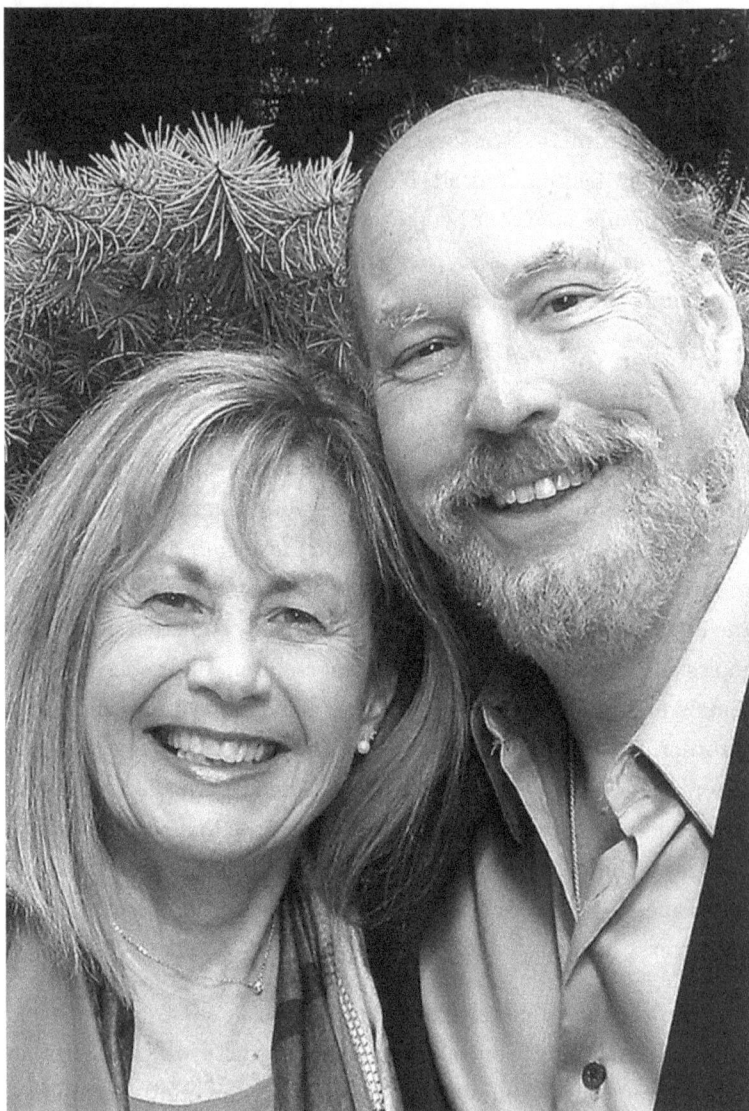

Andi & Jonathan Goldman

CHAPTER 3

HUMMING: *A hum is a sound made by producing a wordless tone with the mouth closed, forcing the sound to emerge from the nose. Humming is producing such a sound.*

YOUR BREATH & HUMMING: CREATING THE VIBRATIONS THAT HEAL

By Andi & Jonathan Goldman

Many years ago, I had a transformational experience when I was on stage in a seaside bar in Marshfield, Massachusetts, in Cape Cod. I was strapping on a guitar looking at the audience when I had an insight about the music that I was creating. Was the music I was making helping to induce an ambience of negativity and violence? The alcohol and the other intoxicants flowing were certainly doing that, but was the music being created adding to that mix? I thought, if music can have this much power, surely it can be used to make people feel better? Surely sound can be used to heal?

This was a revelatory moment for me, after which I dedicated my life to researching sound healing – sharing the information, technique, and processes with others. It wasn't that rock & roll is bad for us per se. It's more about the kind of energy we bring to the music, and the consciousness and desired outcomes of the sound being created.

My partner and wife of over 20 years, Andi, is a holistic psychotherapist who uses expressive therapies in her practice. Not only is she my partner in the journey of life, but also my partner in the sound healing work we do. We have worked together for over 27 years to help people heal holistically using natural therapies including sound, yoga, meditation, pranayama and so on. For her, sound is one of the most expressive of therapies and one that really works powerfully for healing. As Andi says, each of us is a unique vibratory being, and each of us experiences music in a unique, individual manner. We honor all music genres equally and we believe that any music, depending upon the time, the place and the need of the individual, *can* be therapeutic. In fact I once made a presentation on "Blues As Healer" at a major music medicine conference.

I was so strongly convinced about the power of sound that I got a master's degree from Lesley University researching the uses of sound and music for healing. I then founded the Sound Healers Association, and created my record label Spirit Music for therapeutic music. My label has won many awards including a Grammy nomination. I feel so fortunate that Andi and I are able to bring our respective strengths to the table to use sound and breathing techniques to help transform and heal lives. It isn't complicated. It is straightforward, and it is something anyone can do to transform and become empowered.

Sound Healing – How It Works Miracles

There are two ways that sound affects us: psycho acoustics and vibro acoustics. Psycho acoustics can be defined as the process when the sound goes into our ear and into our brain, affecting our nervous system. This then impacts our hardware: heart rate, respiration, brainwaves are all affected on one level by the psycho acoustics.

With vibro acoustics the sound goes directly, physically into our bodies, and affects us at a cellular level, such as when we use tuning forks on our body. A sound bed or sound chair designed to have these specific impacts are other examples of vibro acoustics. These devices are designed to give users a deep harmonizing sound massage, which propels the sound vibration directly into the body. During our research, Andi and I discovered that on a vibro acoustic level, humming is the most powerful vibro acoustic sound and effect that we can create using our own voice. We have developed a specific technique of doing this which we call "Conscious Humming". This has been at the center of our research and work, and I explain why in this chapter.

Therapeutic ultrasound used widely in physiotherapy is another example of sound that helps in the healing process. Here, high frequency sound waves create vibrations and movement of cellular fluids, which is seen to help healing of the body's soft tissues. This works in two ways. Firstly, by stimulating blood flow to the area to promote healing and ease inflammation. Secondly, it helps to stimulate collagen production and help accelerate the healing process in the (injured) tendon and ligament tissue. Studies support this[1] and physiotherapists have been offering this form of therapy for many years now. So what is sound healing and what does it actually entail? Our concept of using Conscious Humming as a modality of sound healing is using single tones that don't really modulate too much with pitch or rhythms. Music is complex and endlessly variable because it has rhythm, melody, harmony, et cetera. So rather than Mozart we work with Tibetan bowls or a tuning fork to create more monotone sounds, and work principally with these sounds to bring about healing.

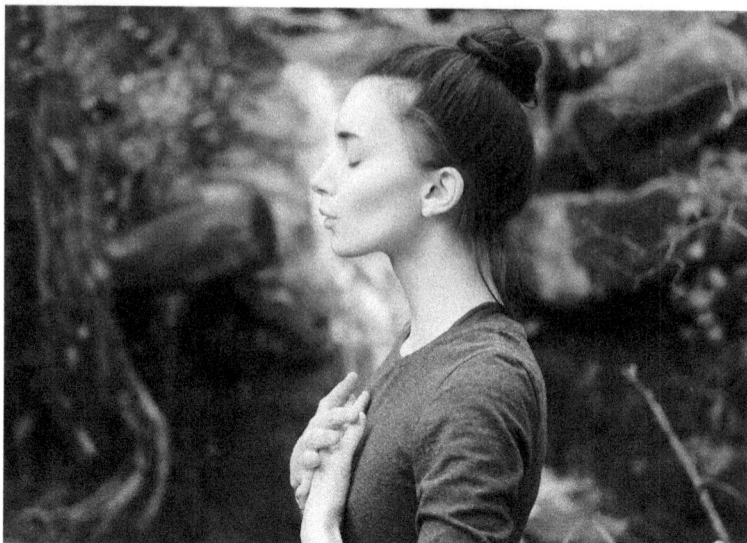

The Importance of Breathing The Right Way

We start to breathe the moment we come out into the world. It isn't something that we have to learn, right? We can't have been doing it wrong all these years after all. Turns out we may have been doing it wrong if we have been breathing via the mouth. There are so many benefits of breathing via the nose: more humid, warmer air, efficient filtration, and increased uptake of oxygen. And when you hum as you breathe via the nose, you could generate up to 15 times more nitric oxide.

As far back as 2006, a study by the Karolinska Institute of Sweden[2] found some remarkable results of nasal breathing. They found that there was 15 times the amount of nitric oxide that is generated in the nasal cavity while humming as opposed to just nasal breathing. The research into the many benefits of increased nitric oxide and the vital importance of this molecule in the system is still ongoing. Increasing levels of nitric oxide are being used therapeutically, for treatment of various viruses and bacteria. More recently a study[3] examined the impact of a nitric oxide nasal spray on COVID patients. It was found that the spray could accelerate the reduction in SARS-CoV-2 RNA load versus a saline spray.

Healing Through Harmonics

To recount a personal anecdote, I was doing a presentation for some doctors in Germany via the International Society for Music Medicine in Germany. I was doing a presentation on vocal harmonics. These are sounds within sounds in a sense. I started out by teaching this one sound, which was a very nasal oriented sound. I said we call this Sonic Dristan (a decongestant drug from before that is largely discontinued now). I said that as a funny metaphor, simply because I had observed through experience that if I made this sound, it would clear up my nasal passages.

We have also seen how chronic sinusitis can be cleared up through certain types of humming. This is now well established and we know because we experienced it and continue to do so. Andi and I have been experiencing first hand and our research has proved how nitric oxide affects literally every organ of the body. It is therapeutic and is also helping us become calmer and more relaxed.

You know how in the movies they say 'just breathe' when someone is trying to calm someone else down? This is with good reason. When we breathe deep – we call them diaphragmatic or belly breaths – and then hum, our blood pressure actually drops dramatically. When we take a few moments to just breathe while in a stressful situation, we can feel ourselves become steadier in body and mind. Those hands stop shaking, the mind clears, and we feel steadier. This is also due, in part, to the nitric oxide being generated and basically the effective spread of oxygen throughout the body. It is incredible; the kind of significant positive impact we can bring about simply by breathing and humming.

Nitric oxide is getting noticed a lot in medical and scientific circles recently, particularly the connection of this molecule to the vagus nerve. We can consciously affect and increase vagal tone, or create the relaxation response by deep breathing and through humming. So here everything is interrelated.

During our training programs, we suggest to people to keep their lips closed when they're humming, and secondly that they hum on any one single note that is comfortable to them. The 2006 Karolinska study had examined different frequencies to see how it would resonate in the nasal cavity. They then settled on one frequency, i.e. 130 hertz or cycles a second. However, we are all unique and different and this varies from person to person. So it is important to find the correct pitch for you, which is usually within your conversational voice. This is why Andi and I are always trying to get people to be in their comfort zone when they are humming.

The Vital Importance of Nitric Oxide

Nitric oxide has come to be recognized as helping to enhance the immune system and improve oxygen delivery in the body, with stress reduction and anti-aging impacts among other things. We can see how the deep breathing and humming helps slow down the heart and promotes relaxation. It relaxes the body by producing hormones like oxytocin, which is the bonding or trust hormone, and this makes us feel better and happier.

There is also strong evidence by Ranje Singh, Ph.D., author of "Self-Healing", to suggest that certain sounds such as humming promote production of the hormone melatonin in the body, and we sleep better as a consequence of this. Melatonin is the body's way of timing its circadian rhythms. This hormone is produced as a response to darkness. However, we are surrounded by artificial lights: home illumination, the ambient light in urban areas, and, of course, our laptops and phones and other devices that continually emit light. Is it any wonder that the body is constantly receiving mixed signals and unable to optimize melatonin production?

Humming helps here as well. If you wake up in the middle of the night, and you can't sleep, try humming. It is a safe and effective form of self-soothing. Babies hum. The elderly hum. Everybody hums. Humming is just a very powerful experience and beneficial habit to create. And unlike say, singing, anyone can hum. It doesn't require electricity or tools, and it is free! Some of us are just rank bad singers, where some of us are good singers but may still be very self-conscious of how we sound. So this can, and does, work for everyone.

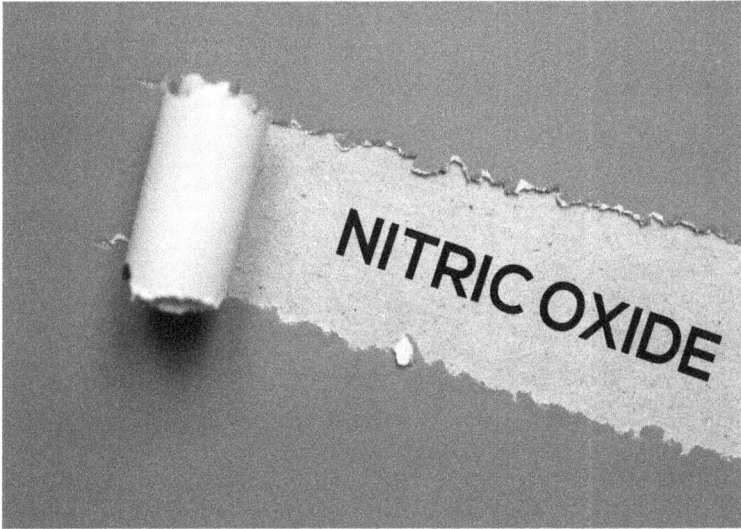

Andi and I have worked with different sounds, mantras, and exercises with chakras and vowel sounds. We have researched quite extensively before deciding that humming is something that people can relate to, and harness the power of what sound can actually do. As we dove deeper into it, we found that yogic traditions also harness the power of the hum.

The profound and powerful yoga technique called *Bhramari pranayama* is one example. This involves very deep breathing and then humming along with certain *mudras* or gestures that cover the face and block the ears. It's still basically the hum, a Conscious Hum. This finds place in the Yoga Sutras by Patanjali – one of the most ancient yogic texts that is thousands of years old. According to Swami Satyananda's translation of it, sutra 1.27 says that the original sound of creation was *prana* or the humming of Om.

We discovered only recently that when we put the tongue right on that little spot, little button behind the front teeth, it helps create that nasalized sound. It brings it more into your nasal cavity and amplifies it further. That same location is also a way of stimulating the pineal gland in yogic traditions. And if you start working with sound and harmonics, it's also a great place to generate these incredible high overtones and nasal harmonics with greater resonance. This is the vibration that really seems to activate nitric oxide production.

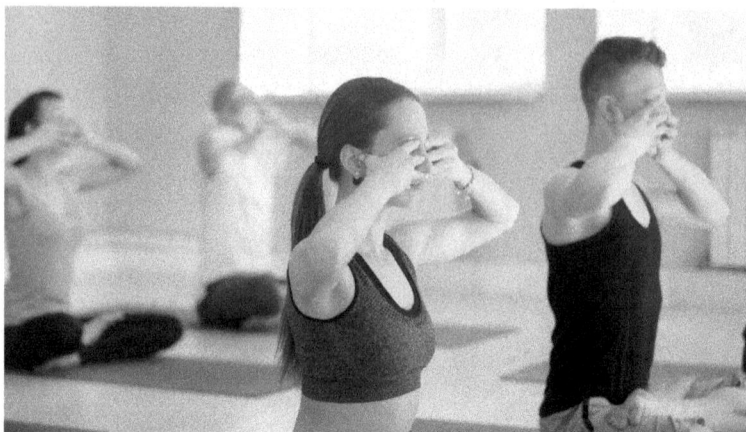

Conscious Nitric Oxide Humming Is Not Humdrum

Andi and I have realized the importance of Conscious Humming for the production of nitric oxide. When we are able to generate the sound to our nose and up to the head, we could, hypothetically, create neurogenesis–the generation of nerve cells in the brain. When we add connections in the brain, through self-created sound and the mechanical resonance, there is reason to believe that neuroplasticity may have a role here. We only have anecdotal information about changing the actual physical brain but serious studies could confirm what we know anecdotally.

So the next question would be, how do we hum, how much and how often?

Well, there are a few things Andi and I have kept in mind to create our protocols. We found that about four or five hums was the maximum level to create peak release of nitric oxide, after which it seems to plateau out. We call this Conscious Nitric Oxide Humming. We then recommend waiting for about three minutes for the cells to regenerate, so that they can again have nitric oxide puffing occur with the sounds that you're making. So we have five hums followed by three minutes of silence, and then five hums again specifically for nitric oxide production. This has a protective impact on health. For people with issues such as chronic sinusitis, an hour's worth of humming with breaks – maybe

15 minutes and then breaking – seems to be very effective. To be clear, more isn't necessarily better, and just humming all day long is not necessary. There is an optimal amount of humming that offers all of the benefits.

That said there could be great personal variations and we are our own best laboratories. We have to discover what works for us. If you have a headache, for example, and you start to hum, and you focus the energy on the headache, and the headache feels better, it is likely that something is going on.

The mother-in-law of a doctor friend of mine had a stroke and some speech impairment. I suggested humming to her and she did it. We didn't see much change on the first or second day, but she sounded better on the third. By day four, she was back to normal. Perhaps it was a coincidence, or perhaps the humming helped?

There is something here for couples as well: in our *Chakra Frequencies: Tantra of Sound*, we have sound exercises for couples to use and to resonate the energy centers. One exercise focuses on the fact that if you're having a disagreement with your partner, the first thing you want to do is use sound.

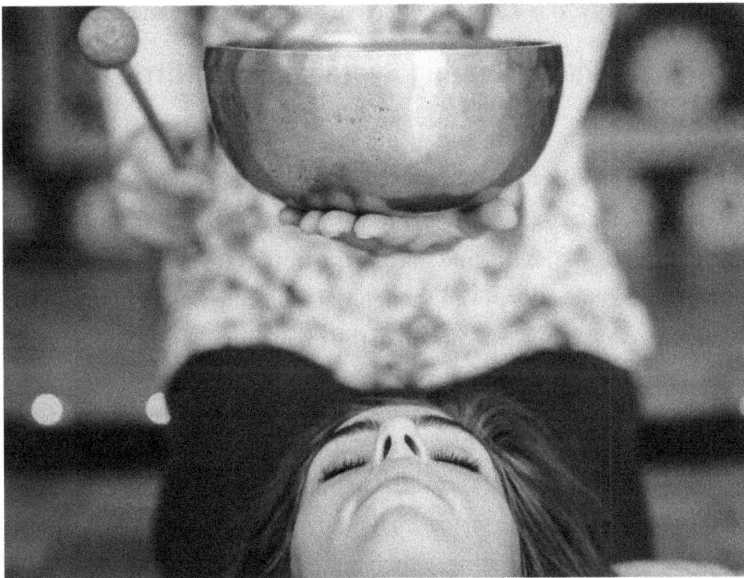

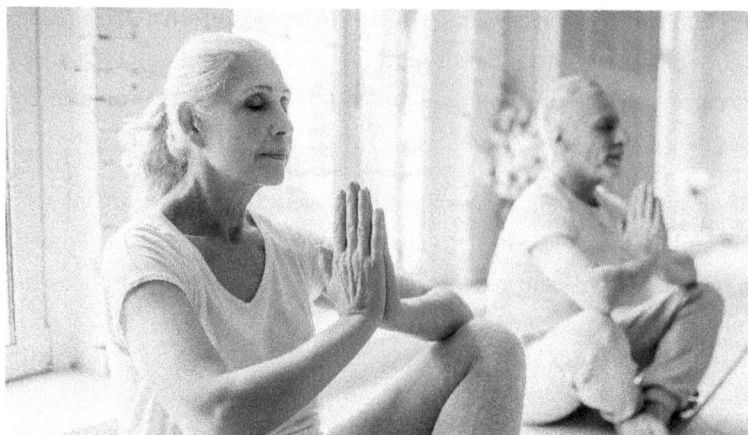

Andi explains this: a disagreement with a partner, child or family member can be resolved by coming together to make a sound. Rather than take it further into the negative energy, she says, "Honey make a sound with me." So we all hold hands even when we don't want to, because we are so mad, but we do it! After a minute or two everything changes – there is a vibrational shift. The mindset changes, the heart and breath rate change. We know that nitric oxide and oxytocin have a role to play here. Soon we're wondering what it was we were so mad about. This actually works as a resolution from a situation that would otherwise degenerate into toxic, hurtful language, and the outpouring of negative energy. It is a simple, effective technique that anyone can use.

How Traditional Healing Systems Used Nitric Oxide

I think that there is a tectonic shift ongoing in the way that western medicine is looking at natural therapies; particularly those that involve nitric oxide. There is some evidence to suggest that traditional or ancient therapy systems understood the importance of humming and nitric oxide generation, even though the molecule wasn't identified as such. The West is now waking up to the many therapeutic applications of this amazing molecule.

We have a beautiful quote from Dr. Bruce Lipton, author of *The Biology of Belief*. He says, "I highly recommend humming for all those impacted by the stress of the modern world. It is a powerful, non-pharmaceutical prescription for self-healing, which has only positive side effects."

The fact that it is non-pharmaceutical could be why this isn't as mainstream as it could be yet. However, I have been working with sound for 40 years, and my wife Andi and I have been working together for 27 years. So we hope to bring more sound healing to the people. As we speak today, it is exploding; being embraced by so many, many, many more people. It is a little like what we saw with yoga a few decades ago when yoga studios cropped up at every corner!

The Seven Secrets of Sound Healing

The 30th anniversary edition of my first book *Healing Sounds* was recently republished with some added new sections. My book *The Seven Secrets of Sound Healing* continues to be widely available and makes sound healing studies accessible and understandable, and also touches on much wisdom and many varied techniques of the healing system that utilizes sound. *The Divine Name: The Sound That Can Change the World*, is another book I've written. This is based on a universal sacred sound composed of harmonically related vowel sounds. It is quite an impressive sonic technology for powerful vibrational healing and transformational experiences. *The Humming Effect* and *Chakra Frequencies* are two of the books that Andi and I have co-authored, which I have spoken of earlier.

I also have over 25 award winning recordings that a great many people throughout the planet have found to be extremely effective for relaxation, stress reduction, meditation and healing. In particular, I would recommend *"Frequencies: Sounds of Healing"* and *"Healing Sounds: Frequencies II,"* both of which feature excerpts from many of these different recordings and both of which have become best sellers.

Our Healing Sounds Intensive is a 10-day program attended by doctors, therapists, and people from all walks of life. We offer a range of programs and training modules on our website healingsounds. com and we are delighted to be sharing our insight and experience with people. The life altering impacts of humming and sound are just tremendous, and someday someone may well win the Nobel when they prove it beyond all doubt!

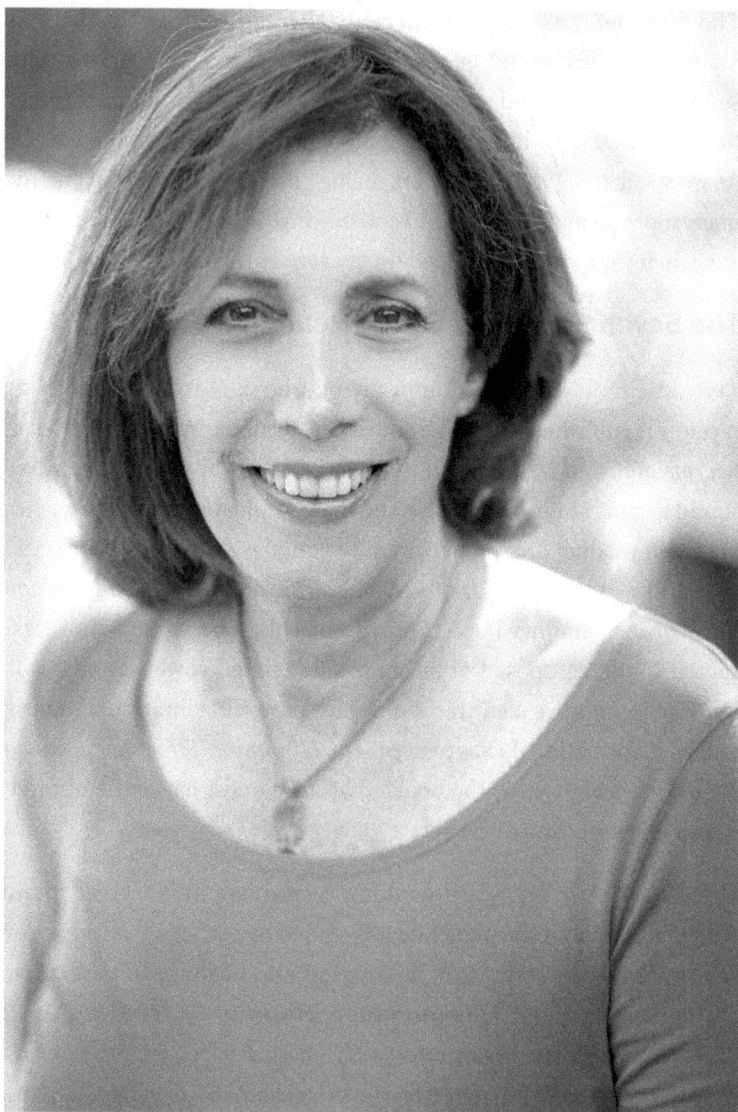

Beth Greer

CHAPTER 4

TOXIC CHEMICALS: *During the manufacturing and use of common products, toxic chemicals are released into the environment. They are absorbed by humans through the skin and nose or ingested in food and water. Up to 300 toxic man-made chemicals have been found in humans – adults and newborns.*

BREATHE IN AND SMELL THE... IS IT CHEMICALS?

By Beth Greer

This was 20 years ago when I was living what I imagined to be a healthy lifestyle. Shoulder pain had me running to the chiropractor. Five treatments did not help and the pain worsened. My first three fingers started to get numb. An MRI revealed a mass in my chest. This was what was pressing on the brachial plexus nerves and causing the pain and numbness. I was forced to examine my 'healthy' life: running a company (The Learning Annex), being stressed all the time, eating out, microwaving my food, no fresh air. Healthy lifestyle? Not so much, I realized.

The tumor biopsy revealed that this wasn't a cancerous mass. However, it was a large nerve root tumor that was causing a lot of pain. Three surgeons wanted to cut me in three different places to access it. This is when I decided that I was going to take charge of my own health. So, going to the Optimal Health Institute, one of the things I was advised to do was to talk to my 'disease'. So I closed my eyes and asked the tumor, *why are you here? What's the message for me?* The answer was – *simplify*. I needed to sort through my complicated life and simplify. I began to look at what I put in me, like food and water; on me, like makeup, soap and shampoo, and things that surrounded me, like household cleaners, scented candles, the air inside my home, and EMFs.

The food ingredient labels were easy, but it started to get complicated when I looked at the stuff I put on my skin. I looked at the label of the moisturizer I used and I saw a paragraph worth of ingredients that I couldn't pronounce. *This can't be good*, was my thought. The skin is our largest organ and all these unidentified ingredients are going right in there. Then I noticed I was cleaning with Windex™, wiping down countertops and other surfaces. The label on the back actually carried a warning about the product being hazardous to humans and domestic animals! And again my thought was *this can't be good*.

I switched to all natural products and I started cleaning with vinegar, white vinegar and hydrogen peroxide. I bought a non-toxic mattress, because the one I had, which was a conventionally made mattress, contained lots of chemicals that were "off-gassing." I also reduced my exposure to EMFs inside my home. I made my bedroom a safe haven in which to sleep and heal.

It took about nine months of uncovering toxins I was exposed to on a daily basis and eliminating them, and then I found that the pain went away. When I underwent another scan, that tumor had disappeared!

Thinking About the Air in Your Body

This was a huge wake-up call for me. I realized that we all have to look very closely at what we put into our bodies, what we surround ourselves with – the air that we breathe 24x7. I put my journalism degree to use and got down to some research. I discovered that in some ways, the air inside our home can be 10 to 20 times more toxic than the air outside, even while living in a city like New York or LA. With all the cleaning products, cosmetics, artificial fragrances, and the indoor mold,

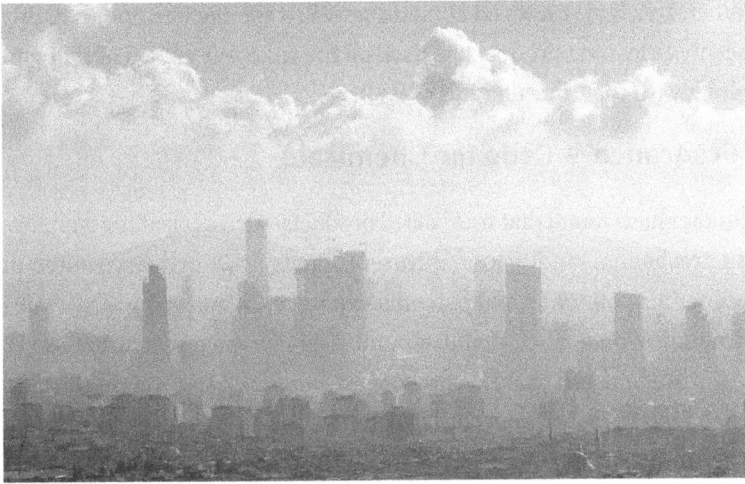

the air we're breathing is actually shockingly polluted. The result of my research and my experiences is my book *Super Natural Home*. It is about our everyday exposure to what can make us ill, and simple suggestions to get healthier.

One of my clients had a chronic cough. She was on codeine cough syrup and an inhaler. Doctors couldn't figure out what was wrong with her. She mentioned to me how when she was in a hotel, she didn't cough. So clearly, something inside her home was responsible for the cough. I walked into her bedroom. She had about 20 scented candles lining her room, and even I could feel my throat starting to get itchy. I told her that this appeared to be the problem. *But these are gifts, they are relaxing, they mean something*, she told me. I convinced her that I put the candles in a bag. Though it was a tug of war, I took them out of her bedroom. I also looked in her medicine cabinet and bathroom, hair products, makeup, nail polish. Everything was scented and took them all out. A few days later, she called me up and she said, *my cough has gone!*

Another example is a woman who ran an organic juice company in San Francisco. She was extremely careful about everything her family ate, making sure it was organic and without sugar, preservatives, artificial colors and so on. However, she, her husband, and her two children had allergies and nothing seemed to help their endless runny noses.

When I visited, I noticed something called the Swiffer 200, a highly scented cleaning product she used all the time. We got rid of that and along with that, the allergies as well!

'Fragrance' – Code for Chemicals

Studies have found that fragranced products, such as cleaning supplies, air fresheners, and personal care products are a primary source of indoor air pollutants and personal exposure.[1] When you see the word 'fragrance' on a label, that is an umbrella term manufacturers use to gloss over the fact that there would be a hundred to several thousand chemicals in there. It may be legal, but it is also very misleading. When you think about the chemicals in candles, shampoo and makeup...it adds up to a lot of chemical exposure. Most of us are exposed to literally thousands of chemicals on a daily basis. Quite simply, our bodies don't know what to do with all of that.

The term 'fragrance' is used to refer to a bunch of chemicals made in a factory and they can disrupt our endocrine system.[2] These are toxic to the upper respiratory systems. This can be deceptive because 'fragrance' is found in so many things, like trash bags, kitty litter, feminine hygiene products. One has to become a detective to know what is really going into the products we use each day. Trash night in my neighborhood doesn't smell like trash anymore. It smells 'nice' because people are using scented garbage bags.

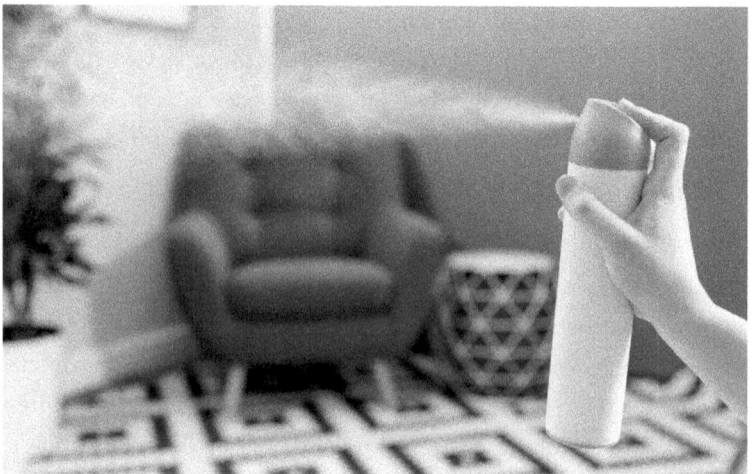

Another product that can be really toxic is dryer sheets. People use them to make the laundry smell nice, but this is a smell that lingers and the fragrance is carried out into the street. When something lasts so long, lingers from your dryer out into the street, you really have to think about how unhealthy that is for you.

I understand that we want our laundry to smell nice but do we really want all those chemicals in our clothes, on our skin, wafting into our airways, getting into our bloodstream? So here's a trick I use: I sprinkle a few drops of lavender essential oil onto a washcloth and throw that into my dryer. That is my dryer sheet essentially, and the clothes come out smelling fantastic: like fresh lavender, but without the chemicals.

Mold – The Enemy Hiding in Plain Sight

Over time, I've become something of a toxin detective. I've gotten used to ferreting out all the different ways in which we ingest toxins: absorption through the skin, inhalation, just exposure of any sort. When it comes to smelling what we breathe, it isn't just fragrances – mold is a huge problem as well. It is far more prevalent than we thought it to be. Studies also show that the negative impacts of mold inhalation on health could be a lot worse than we believed earlier.[3]

One of my clients asked me to come to her home because she was feeling sick and achy. When I did, I smelled the mold right away. She didn't, but this is because of something called olfactory fatigue or adaptation (where we don't smell something after prolonged exposure to a particular airborne compound). The fact is that mold may be lurking where you cannot see or smell it. This woman had wall to wall carpeting. When we had the dust from her vacuum cleaner examined in the lab – an evaluation anyone can have made for about a hundred dollars – it detected very high volumes of mold. She moved out of that toxic environment and quickly healed.

There are a few warning signs to look out for with mold infestations. Condensation on the windows, mold in the top of the toilet tank or in the air conditioning duct could be signs of poor air quality. To prevent mold buildup, it is important to open up the windows from time to time, and clean the HVAC filters regularly.

While some of us can move out of a house with mold, many of us don't have that option. A mold mediator is a good option if things are serious and one's health is involved. Sometimes it is possible to move upstairs while the lower floor is being treated. A lot of the time, upper floors that receive more sunlight may not have a mold problem. The fogging that mold exterminators do can also be a problem since that often involves more toxic chemicals being sprayed into the house. Another problem is that these fogging services tend to be very expensive. It is possible to use mold remediation services that use natural solutions that aren't very expensive either. Haven Cleaning and Restoration is one such service that I have seen to be affordable and effective. (https:// supernaturalmom.com/resources/recommended-products/#mold)

VOCs Can Do What?

In another instance, I had a client who only ate organic food. She made her own almond milk, and would only use natural products on her skin and for cleaning her home. She called me because she had terrible headaches. I asked how long she had been having them, and she said, *17 months*. That was a long time and also quite precise. *So what happened 17 months ago?* This was when she remodeled her home, and put down new carpeting and wallpaper. She didn't see the connection but I could. I could *smell* it. I explained that all this furniture and the new carpeting was emitting all these fumes: the paint, the glue, and so on. A couple of strong air purifiers, and opening the windows to let the stale air out and fresh air in made all the difference.

We are talking about these toxins we inhale – volatile organic compounds. VOCs have a distinctive plastic-like smell. Traditional furniture would often be sprayed with toxic flame retardants. Now thanks to laws passed, you can choose products that haven't been treated with flame retardants.

The Detox Process

Exposure to toxins could cause a buildup in the body. So should we detox? How can we detox? A lot of the time, the toxins in our body will be eliminated gradually when we remove the source of those toxins.

Change the cleaning materials, personal care products, ventilate the home, call in a mold remediation service, and things tend to clear up. The great thing about the human body is that with proper hydration, nutrition, and quality supplements, the body will restore itself most of the time. I find that activated charcoal can help. The important thing is to stop the toxic assault; to remove the body from exposure to the toxins.

Having a few indoor plants also helps. It is best to have plants in the living room and office areas, and even the bathrooms and the kitchen. I personally don't like plants in the bedroom because of the carbon dioxide they emit during the night hours. The thing to watch out for here is to not have too many plants because you then run the risk of moldy soil, condensation in the windows, and so on. So, there are an optimal number of plants you can have in the home for the benefits you can derive. I find that a couple of plants in each room is ideal. Some plants are good for getting rid of benzene and certain plants are good for absorbing formaldehyde.

When you're buying products, one of the things to watch out for is *greenwashing*. They label something 'green' or 'herbal' or 'natural' but this may not be strictly accurate. Some of the time, the only natural thing may be the biodegradable packaging. The contents may still be full of chemicals, fragrance, artificial colors and so on.

During the lockdown, I was working out of my home for a long time, managing with my phone and laptop. During this time, I helped a woman in Connecticut who was having terrible headaches. It turned out that she had an alarm system in her house that was on all the time that was the culprit. When she turned it off, her headaches went away!

It is also sometimes the case that one of two people living in the home is reacting badly to something – cleaning products or mold for instance. We are genetically all different and each of us will react differently to the same stimuli. So, maybe we all need to become toxin detectives! You really don't know what you could be inhaling or absorbing that is causing you to become ill.

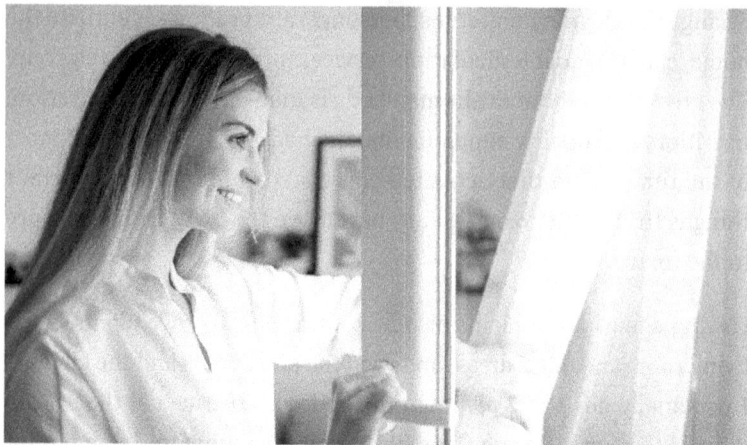

Open The Windows

While it isn't possible to leave the windows open all the time, try to do this for an hour or so every day. It may not be possible to turn off the AC and open the windows in the afternoon but maybe you could do this during the cooler parts of the day. It is a good idea to get out and into nature at dawn. The fresh air, the sound of the birds, and the sun hitting the eyes and the skin is great for us. We know that the gradual lightening of the sky has a positive impact on our natural circadian rhythms, and just the fresh air does us a world of good. We can walk, run, hike, cycle, meditate, sit on a park bench listening to a podcast, or just enjoy some quiet time. Taking the time to be out in nature is something that I do consciously; particularly after the tumor incident all those years ago.

Modern lifestyles have given rise to something known as the nature-deficit disorder, particularly among kids. Being indoors all the time takes a toll on physical, mental, and emotional well-being, as we have seen particularly during the COVID pandemic. Kids that spend more time in green spaces are seen to have lower stress, better attention spans, and more positive feelings.[4] The 'stay on the trail' instructions, or the 'look don't touch' signs, the parental desire to keep kids indoors for their safety...all this has meant kids living lives unnaturally cut off from natural outdoor environments. Today's kids aren't being allowed to do the sort of things older generations simply took for granted.

Taking Care of Indoor Air

We make the mistake of thinking about the outside air as polluted and indoor air as safe. Actually in the last several years, there has been a growing body of scientific evidence that the air within homes and other buildings can be more seriously polluted than the outdoor air.[5] Since most of us spend 90% of our time indoors, the risks to health from indoor air pollution may be very significant.

For cleaning, white vinegar and water works for a lot of cleaning requirements. You can often find gentle, non-toxic products at Whole Foods or Trader Joes. There is a recommended product list at my website supernaturalmom.com. Basically go for things that are gentle and unscented; that have a short list of ingredients vis-à-vis a ton of unpronounceable chemicals.

A lot of the time, the good old wet mop may be the best way to trap and get rid of the indoor dust that can cause allergies and respiratory issues. Using HEPA filters in the home's HVAC system or the vacuum cleaner is another important way to get rid of indoor pollutants. Use these simple but important ways to control the air you breathe, and the things that your skin absorbs.

Remember all of us don't react the same way to the same products. That doesn't mean that someone's illness or suffering isn't just as real. Be a toxin detective. Examine all of the things that you breathe in, put on your skin, or that you use around the house. By process of elimination, see what it is that doesn't agree with you.

The solutions that you seek may actually be simple and easy to find. The toxins could be right there, hiding in plain sight. They could be fumes from paint or glue or flame retardants, the 'fragrance' in your hygiene products or makeup, mold that lurks in corners of your home, or even an electronic alarm system! My recommended non-toxic household products, EMF radiation protection, non-toxic personal care and makeup, as well as supplements are listed on supernaturalmom.com. Who knows, making small changes could mean that you could improve your health and even avoid surgery as I did.

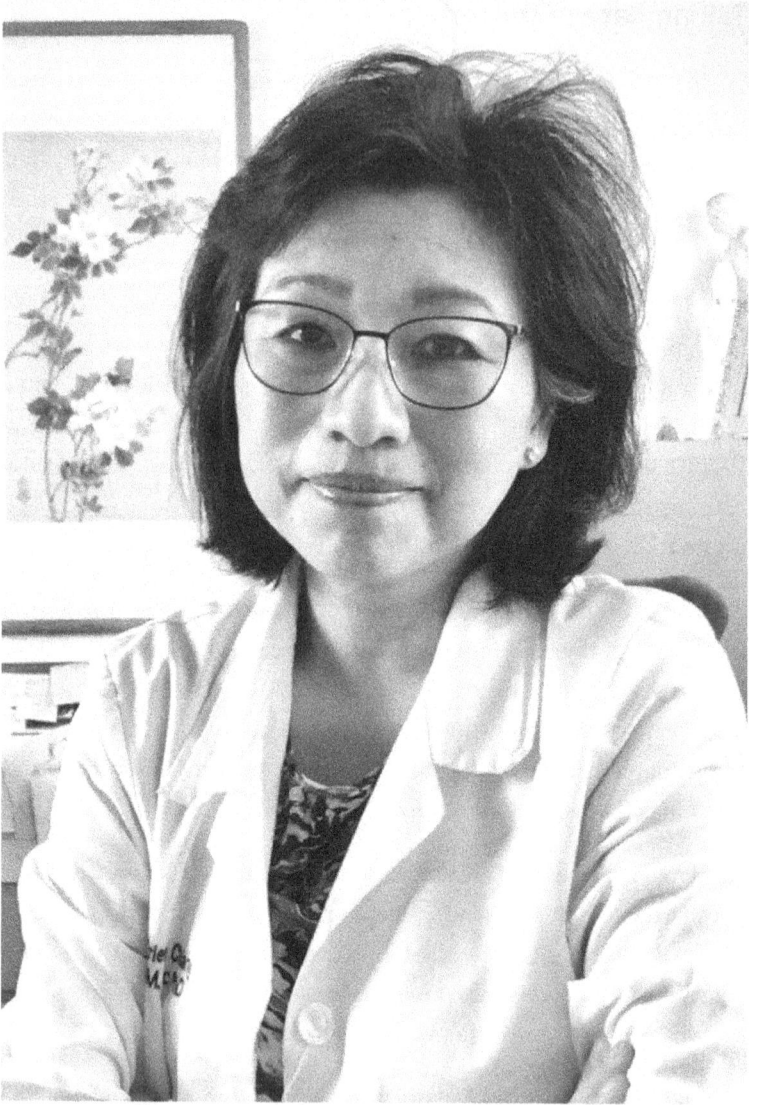

Dr. Erlene Chiang

CHAPTER 5

QIGONG: *(pronounced chi gong) was developed many centuries ago in China as part of traditional Chinese medicine. It involves using exercises to optimize energy within the body, mind, and spirit, with the aim of improving and maintaining health and well-being.*

THE ART OF BREATHING: AS IMPORTANT TODAY AS IT WAS IN ANCIENT CHINA

By Dr. Erlene Chiang

As someone who straddles the dual world of traditional Chinese and modern Western medicine, I like to bring a holistic perspective to health, well-being, and healing. I find that many of the same principles of good health that the ancients spoke about are reflected and reinforced by our modern understanding of the human body. The centrality of breathing in our life, and its importance for our health and well-being is one of those principles.

One of the earliest known textbooks of Chinese medicine is the *Huangdi Neijing* (The Yellow Emperor's Inner Classic). By the 4th and 6th century, Chinese philosophers such as Lao Tzu and Chuang Tzu were already speaking about breathing – the inhale and the exhale. They were speaking about the exchange of information in Daoism, of practice in a guided direction. Books on Qigong, dating back to the 4th and 6th century period, speak about the ancient methods of breathing. It is believed that people used to live for 120 years on average in those times. The fact that people now die at age 50 or 60, even as early as 30 or 40, is possibly because of a new mutation. People aren't taking care of themselves, we are seeing more cancer and genetic diseases, and people are dying early because of these genetic reasons.

People followed nature back in the day. They followed Yin and Yang. The Yin is like in the nighttime quietness, while Yang is active sunlight. People used to follow the sun: when the sun came out, they got up, exercised, went outside, stretched, and started working. Evening time is when people and their biological systems become naturally quiet, calm down, and then go into rest mode or sleep mode. So do the plants and the animals that also have this biological rhythm; it is what we see all around us. For instance, rice is grown in the spring and summertime, and harvested and stored in the fall and winter time. Following nature is fundamental to life. By reversing this you cannot preserve your well-being and your vitality.

And what does this have to do with breathing? Breathing is our most fundamental activity. It is what you do when you are first born. The first thing you did when you came out as a little baby was to breathe. The first thing a doctor does is to check if the baby is breathing. So breathing is fundamental; nutrition and food are secondary.

Breathing, Longevity, and The Concept Of Qi

Healthy people who live a long life are the ones who have a regular rhythm, regular diet, and regular lifestyle. They get up early, they go to bed at about the same time each day, eat healthy, and they keep their body and their mind healthy and quiet, which is the reason they can prolong their life. It is the job of Chinese healers to try to keep a healthy balance between the Yang (active) and Yin (passive) forces within the human body. When this balance is harmonious and in order, the person enjoys sound physical health. On the other hand, disturbance or interruption of this balance results in illness or disorder in the body.

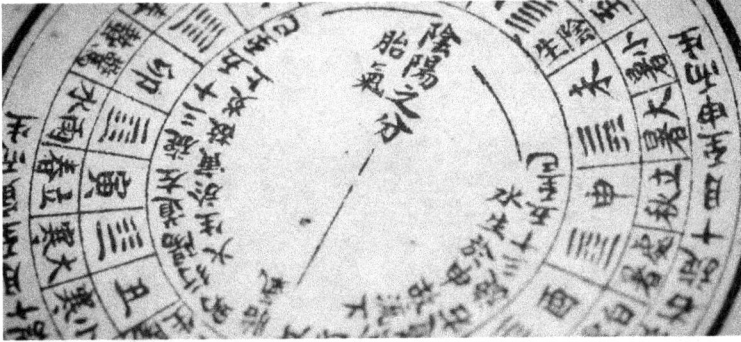

To find the reasons for their health and longevity, I often look at some of my patients. There are instances where the grandmother has cancer and the mother has cancer, but the kid doesn't have cancer. We see how cancer skips a generation and then the following generation has cancer again – why is this? What did this person do right – or wrong? Traditional Chinese medicine has some of the answers, as does Qigong. Qi, or chi as some people spell it, is our life force. It is something we all are born with; we call it the original source.

At birth, the body has the building blocks for a long and healthy life: breathing, organ function, cell division, then brain development. With good nutrition, we reach our physical potential at about 20 or 25 years of age. Breathing is a big part of this. That is the original source Qi, the concept that has been handed down for some 2000 years. From this emerges the concept of Qigong – literally 'life energy cultivation'.

What Is Qigong?

Qigong is the traditional Chinese system that has its roots in Chinese traditional medicine, philosophy, and martial arts. It consists of coordinated movements and body postures that also combine meditation and breathing techniques. The system has applications in spirituality and health, as well as martial arts training. One form of this discipline is called wild goose Qigong, which is about 1800 years old and is still being taught today. Additionally there are 10 other (11 in all) Qigong forms approved by the Chinese government department of physical health based on its authenticity, originality, and medical efficacy.

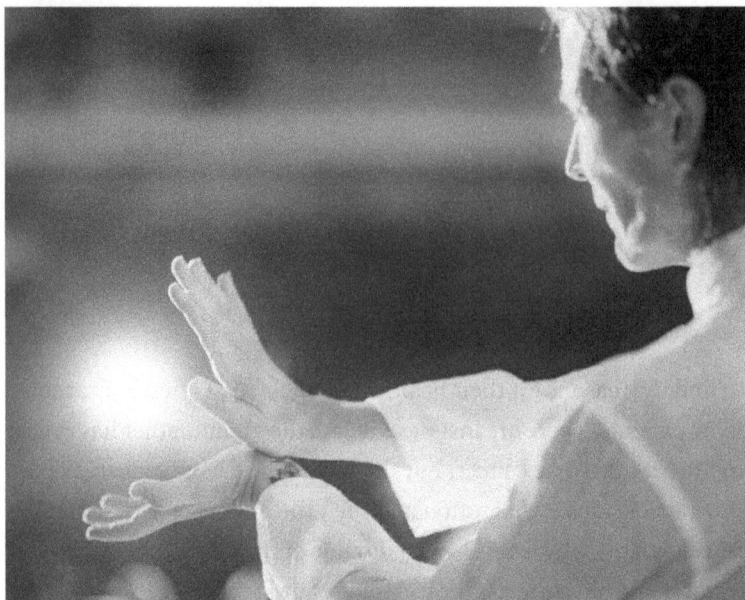

In China, where Qigong first started, there are millions of practitioners. They're practicing Qigong, practicing breathing, practicing that transformation to reach the full potential for good health and long life. Studies have shown the many positive outcomes among Qigong practitioners.[1] Several randomized, controlled trials showed that many health parameters saw significant improvements as a result of practicing Qigong. This included health aspects such as bone density, cardiopulmonary effects, physical function, and reduction of falls and related risk factors. The studies also examined quality of life, self-efficacy, patient reported outcomes, psychological symptoms, and immune function, which also saw positive correlations.

Most of us don't breathe the right way nowadays. We aren't trained or taught. We don't practice breathing the way we should and we don't have the habit of breathing the right way. We lose the natural rhythm of breathing. If you watch a baby breathing – that baby doesn't have conscious thoughts; food, air and love is all they need. When you watch a baby breathing, you see that they never breathe shallowly. They breathe deep, they sleep deeply and calmly – they sleep like a baby! Their breath is calm, the inhale and exhale are all very rhythmic and natural.

Now contrast this with people that have asthma or COPD or any lung impairment or obstruction. They can no longer breathe normally. Along with the body's lung function, the heart function, the circulatory system, and the metabolic function becomes damaged and impaired. It is important to clear the original source, to clear the air, which is the original foundation. Without air there is no Qi, and without that there is no life force. When your Qi is not aligned, the food you eat will not have that transformational ability. The oxygen in the air you breathe is unable to be carried by the blood effectively to the cells of the body.

Qigong and Breathing

In this system of movement, the lungs expand horizontally and vertically, from the front and the back. The apex of lungs rises almost to the collarbones and expands all the way across with the bottom of the lungs expanding all the way down to the diaphragm. This helps expand the capacity of the lungs and helps us to breathe better.

Traditional systems such as tai chi, Qigong, yoga, and meditation are soft and gentle physical activities. There is no age limitation and no physical limitation. With harder, rigorous physical activities like jogging, swimming, team or contact sports, there could be certain limitations and contraindications. These activities may not be suitable for older people, or people with impairments or mobility issues. However, tai chi, yoga, and Qigong, which consist of stretching and other ancient exercises, are suitable for everyone.

Qigong and tai chi practices follow the nature of the Yin and the Yang, as I mentioned above. This means that the stretching, the different positions, and each extension of the movement can be adapted to different requirements. It doesn't require specific fixed practice. It is all very soft and slow, which doesn't require a lot of rigorous effort or movements that are difficult to perform for the body. All through this, breathing is very essential. Air is very essential. With the soft movement, this comes naturally. You don't have to sit and practice breathing because your physical and lung movement has already helped coordinate your breath. Your body is very intelligent that way. If you feed your body good food, and give it access to energy sources, the body

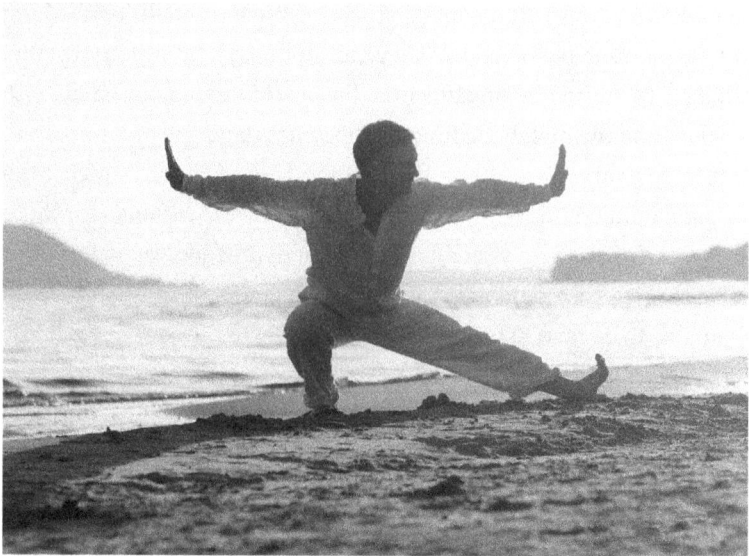

can do exactly what it needs to regulate itself. The body makes room for the breath that comes into the body. It opens up in an optimal way along with those movements.

How The Body Gets Polarized, and How to Restore Balance

Why do we get ill? Why do we have acute or chronic conditions? Maybe this is because of not breathing enough. Maybe it is because the mind and brain are separated. Anxiety, a sedentary life, and poor lifestyle habits can all cause sickness. In traditional medicine, healing consists of 30% treatment and 70% nurturing. Nurturing is meditation, gentle exercise; it is regulating sleep timings, and bringing harmony to the body by being active, eating well, and reducing anxiety. All of these help to banish sickness and improve longevity. However, when illness and imbalance continue, when anxiety and stress become routine, this is when the body becomes polarized. This could manifest in sickness, even cancer. In Chinese medicine, when the body is polarized the organs no longer function properly, the cells malfunction, inflammation occurs, and things go haywire.

Qigong books say this, as do researchers: the Qi emitted from the hand is between eight to twelve hertz. All the different sources of electricity around us, the internet and so on, interfere with the body's electric circuit. The wiring, the radiation that comes in from the appliances, the gadgets, Wi Fi, high speed internet, and a phone tower are never very far from us. All this interferes and interacts with the system. The body starts to be deviated because of this. If you lead a regular disciplined life in the Blue Zone, this doesn't matter. If not, things start to go awry.

We developed artificial intelligence, and people became so intelligent, they forgot and lost their natural rhythm! They became deviated and ill. So these are some of the things that we need to revisit.

Longer Life or Quality of Life?

When we think about health and longevity, one of the things to keep in mind is quality of life. The medical community tends to concentrate more on prolonging life than on enhancing it. Maybe we live longer than the generation before us, but if we're doing this while popping endless pills, or living with pain and dysfunction, is that even worth our while? When they prescribe medications, are they even trying to weed out the root cause of disease, or are they taking care of just the symptoms?

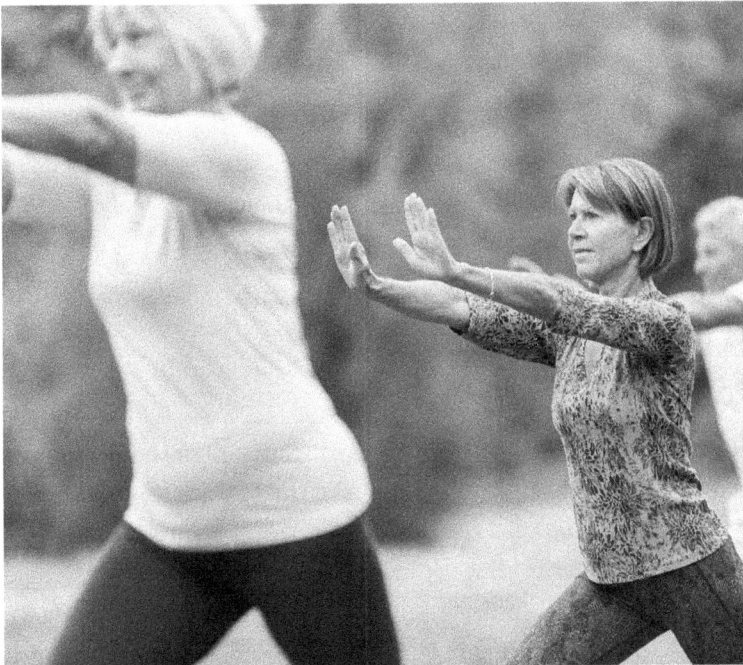

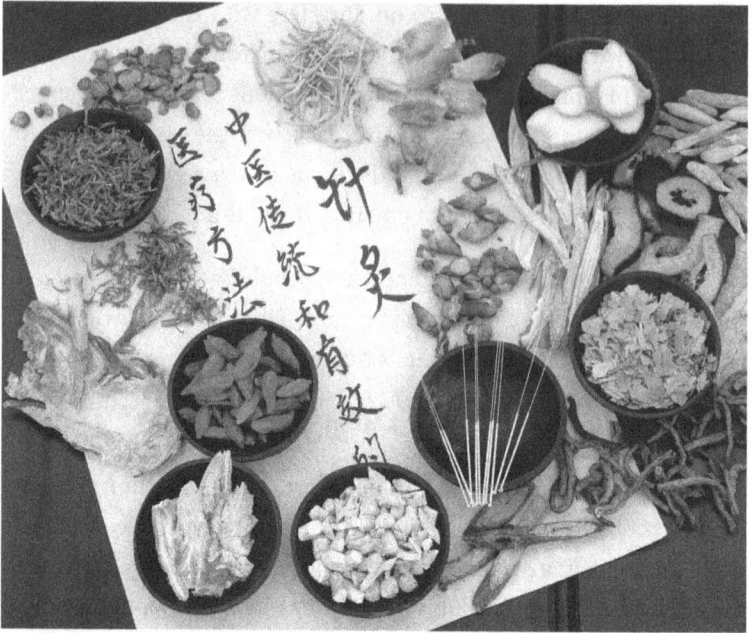

We spend billions on fixing the symptoms, not the disease. And this is why we need to look at the components of the body, and try to restore balance, regularity, and rhythm. We must aim to surround ourselves with love and care of dear ones because this nourishment of the soul is as important as food.

We must aim for wholesome homemade nutrition, produced from the earth, touched by the sun – that is as close to its natural state as possible. We must aim to listen to the wisdom of our body. Yes, we must make use of technology to be healthier and fitter, but not to the point that it interferes with our well-being and our precious balance.

Science and Tradition – Complementary Or Clashing?

Right now in the West there is no way to measure the body's Qi, and the scientific method cannot yet be applied to the wisdom of the natural body's health. Who knows, we will soon be able to do this as well. There are already studies ongoing in China, Taiwan, and Japan, where Qigong is widely prevalent. In these Asian countries tai chi, and the balance of Yin and Yang is common. Perhaps the United States is yet to catch up but we're making progress. For the past 25 years, San Francisco, Toronto, and other parts of the world have been hosting the World Congress of Qigong. Scientists come from all over the world to present their discoveries, to debate what we can see, what is real. Can you see air? Can you not see air? Can you see pollution? Can you see clean air? We cannot. So why do we doubt that Qi exists simply because we cannot see it – yet? In a closed room, you can feel stuffy but you cannot see the stuffiness. When you go out, you can feel and smell the fresh air but you cannot see it.

The National Institutes of Health are delving into this and studies are being conducted on this subject. After all, what is the differentiation, and can science say something conclusively one way or the other? The simple answer is, not yet.

Take acupuncture for instance. We have the different meridians of the body as traditional Chinese medicine understands it. We also have the different acupuncture points that we target to free up trapped Qi within the body to help restore balance. When we draw blood at specific points, such as the lungs, large intestines and so on, the blood work shows higher levels of calcium, magnesium, or iron at some of those points. So clearly there is some scientific rationale behind the targeting of those specific points.

We have also seen how stimulating acupuncture points in an fMRI setting causes parts of the brain to light up. We have seen how this stimulation helps in improving bowel function, reducing inflammation, and increasing energy or functions. Researchers at the NIH and elsewhere in the world continue to examine the energy pathways in the body, and try to see how they correspond to the body's meridians and the body's Qi.

Now it is true that life as we know it would be impossible without modern science. But does this mean that we abandon traditional knowledge systems? Do we cast out ancient wisdom and deprive ourselves of its intuitive insight? Chinese medicine has been around for 3000 years, and the fact that it is still alive helps answer these questions. The smartphone we use now is a far cry from the device we

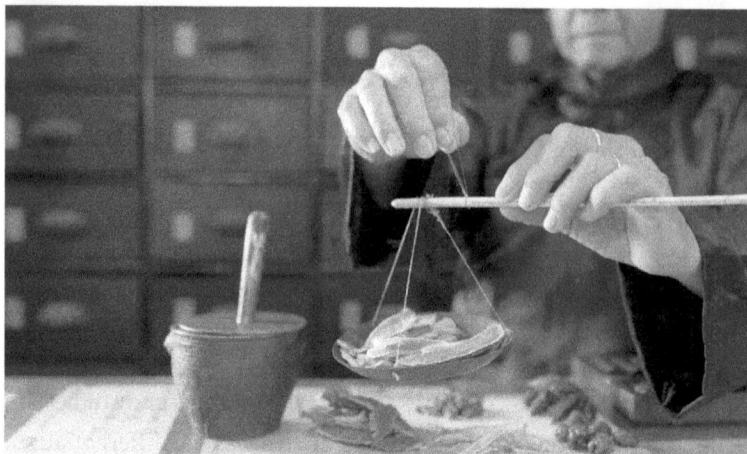

used ten years ago. We didn't abandon that technology; merely built on it, refined it, and improved it. That intelligence and that wisdom was then enhanced as we went along. In the same way, the traditional and the modern can coexist and complement each other.

Humility is important. Dismissing tradition as primitive or unrefined would be a mistake, because we then deprive ourselves of the collective wisdom of some of the finest minds of the last few thousand years.

Circling Back to Breathing

While I am a Chinese traditional medicine practitioner, acupuncturist, and Qigong teacher, a majority of my work is actually in oncology or cancer treatment and care. Sometimes I am called on to deal with patients at the very last stage of their life with a couple of days, maybe a week left. When I work with such individuals, I teach them how to breathe; I educate the family. Why do I do that? At this stage, the patient's on a lot of morphine or narcotic pain meds, and the patient is already like a zombie. The family is very worried, the patient is dying, and it's a terrible situation that the healthcare provider is dealing with.

The patient's breathing is very shallow at this point, and the heartbeat may be as high as 100 to 120 or even 140. No medicine will really slow it down. However, I sit next to this patient with very rapid breathing, a high heart rate, and I practice heavy breathing to make my heart rate climb as well. I match their breathing and their tone. I have to be very focused and I find that I get into a meditative state at such times. And then I use my breath to slow down theirs – it is empathetic, a natural power like a caring hug. We all have this power, but we tend to forget it. We are so wrapped up in technology that we forget to utilize this inner power of ours.

To give yourself a demo, do this: stand up and try this basic warmup exercise – some arm rotations with the arms locked. You then push up from your arm and your wrist and you feel your whole body pushing up and forward a bit. Now take a deep breath and you will feel how that helped open you up from the inside. There is just more room for the air to flow into the body.

Now stretch up with the arms up towards the ceiling, and let the ribcage open up. The shoulders, the armpits all open up, and you can just breathe better. Even in a seated position, you can go back and open up the ribcage to breathe more and better. Relax your shoulders and breathe in while engaging your diaphragm. This targets the joints and the connective tissue, what we call the meridians, to allow more air in. It improves posture and the oxygenation of the organs. This also gives the organs more space to function better and in a less constricted space.

Give yourself the chance to experience better health; to live life not just longer, but more fully, with the simple expedient of breathing better. The Chinese ancients knew this, thousands of years ago – why not take advantage of this now, today, and change your life for the better?

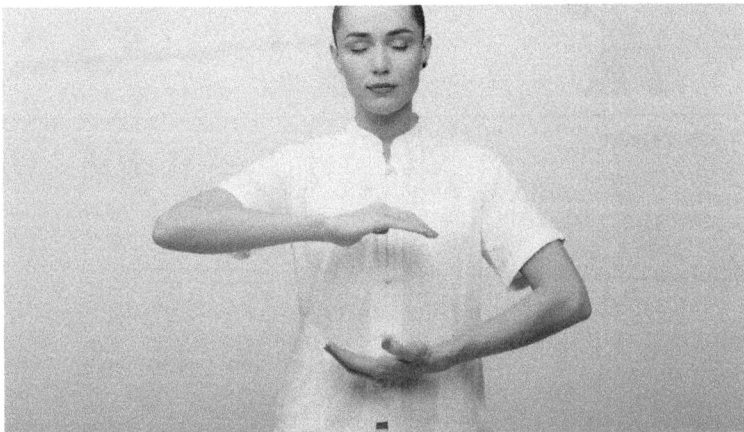

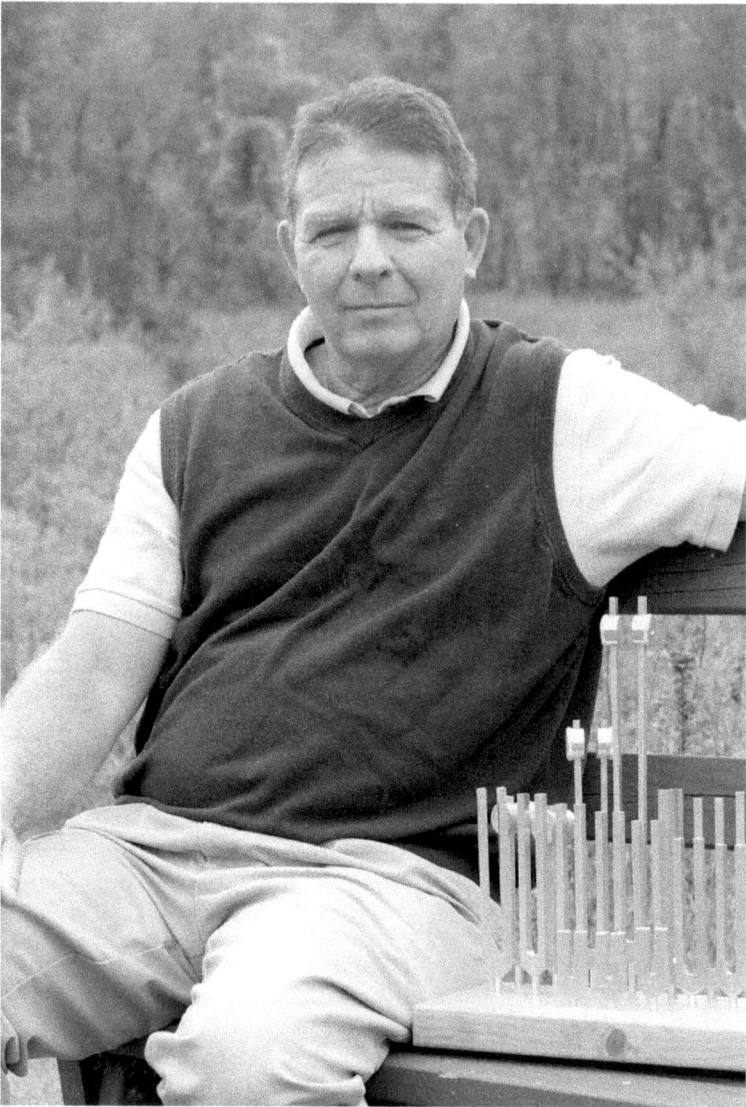

Dr. John Beaulieu

CHAPTER 6

SOUND HEALING: *Sound healing is the practice of using sound and listening in a mindful manner to transform and expand consciousness in order to enhance the body's natural drive to regenerate and heal itself. Sound healers use instruments like gongs, singing bowls, and tuning forks, to relax your mind and body to relieve stress, reduce anxiety, and help with sleep disorders.*

SOUND, BREATH, AND THE COHERENCE OF OUR NERVOUS SYSTEM

Dr. John Beaulieu

To explain how we create sound, and how sound affects us and our well-being, let me explain with a personal anecdote. I was hired by New York University in 1973 as a clinical research psychologist at Bellevue Psychiatric Hospital in New York. In the corner of my laboratory there was a small room on wheels, called an anechoic chamber. This is a chamber designed by engineers that is totally silent and dark. It is like a desensitization chamber that was put there in the 1950s by the CIA. It has been abandoned for many years. Psychologists most likely conducted interrogation experiments using LSD. I knew what it was and I was able to use it to conduct sound experiments. I would sit in the anechoic chamber and listen to the sounds my own body was making. I meditated on the sounds of my body and kept a journal of my experiences. I was doing Phenomenological Research.

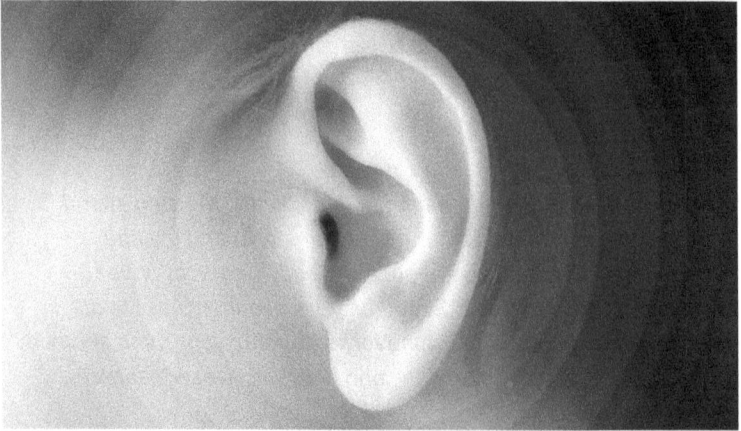

One day on my way to work I got into an argument with the subway toll booth attendant. I didn't realize how much that argument had affected me until I got back into my lab and sat in the anechoic chamber. Usually when I went into the anechoic chamber, I would hear the sound of the nervous system as a high pitch, which was the high sound of my nervous system functioning. However, this time when I went into the anechoic chamber my nervous system sound was loud, jarring, pounding, and screaming. I was shocked and could not understand it. I had been walking around for about 45 minutes with my nervous system like this – with these jangling, discordant sounds within me? I didn't even know it? That is what really shocked me!

I got to thinking about how this state impacted my health and well-being without me not even being aware of it. The silence, isolation, and sensory deprivation of the anechoic chamber was the reason I became aware. This is when I realized that I was "out of tune" and needed to tune myself. I ran downstairs to a music store and I purchased two tuning forks – a C and a G. I tapped them on my knees and brought them to my ears. They had an instant impact on my nervous system. I immediately experienced being unified, and a deep feeling of calmness and silence. I went from being exceedingly stressed to centered and serene in a matter of moments. So what had happened? It was just sound, not even music, just sound. The experience was simple and profound, and it is something that I have been researching and talking and writing about for almost 50 years.

What Is Sound Healing?

My experiences in the anechoic chamber showed me that there were definitely healing properties in sound – in the vibrations sounds produce, and the impacts these have on our body and brain. While music is said to transcend cultures, sound does this even more effortlessly. Consider how, someone from India may find reggae music less accessible or appealing than someone from the Caribbean. Similarly, the sound of an operatic tenor may sound inscrutable to someone from a traditional African culture vis-à-vis someone born and brought up in Italy.

So while music is a global language, certain natural sounds are even more so. Sounds like the crashing of the waves on the shore or a gurgling brook, the chirping of birds or the sound of the breeze through the branches of a tree are universally identifiable. The sound of falling rain, a small child's unbridled laughter, or the crunch of fresh snow underfoot – these are all beautifully evocative.

Sounds can be jarring or soothing. We know that because we experience this every day. For instance, the sound of a snarling dog can be terrifying, but the happy yip of a dog could mean warm cuddles for someone else. The sound of traffic can be stressful, and the vibrations of motor vehicles can be exhausting, while the sound of the wind rushing across the face while riding a bike briskly can be exhilarating.

It is clear that sound has some very specific impacts on our mood, emotions, and feelings. So I began listening to and experimenting with the sounds of tuning forks. I had recorded the C & G and other tuning intervals and listened to them on special headphones called the Bone Fone. A Bone Fone hangs around your neck and under your shirt, and vibraties the sounds of the tuning forks through bone conduction. I even listened while I was sleeping.

I immersed myself in the sounds of different tuning fork intervals, i.e., C & G, C & F, C & A, for 24 hours a day. I was a little crazy about it. I suppose everything was a bit extreme back in the 70s. I did tone it down after a point, but remained convinced of the power of sound healing. I also became aware of the importance of breathing, the sound of it, and the way it integrates into the practice of healing.

Integrating Breathing With Sound

There are specific sounds and tones that keep us feeling unified, coherent, and centered, whether it is the tuning forks, or even the sound of our breathing or ourselves humming. It doesn't matter if you don't have tuning forks. You can just close your eyes, pretend you have them, and hum their tone. With some practice you will find that you can self-regulate, and do this whenever you feel the need to manage stress or navigate a difficult situation. You can do this tuning fork practice with a C and G tuning fork anytime and anywhere.

We can work with sound and with breath to really make a change. When we experience stress, rather than sitting there and fighting it, we must listen to it, meditate with it. The scientific community is in agreement about the importance of the molecule nitric oxide for good health, and how the flatlining or diminishing of nitric oxide is associated with many diseases (more about this below in this chapter).

While I was experimenting in the anechoic chamber I realized that I was breathing using my upper chest. When I listened to the sound of C & G, I felt my whole breath go down to my my belly and then back up into my chest. So once we're in a state of coherence, our breath finds its own way. I combined breath and sound very effectively in this way.

The 5-second breath is really simple. You breathe in for five seconds, you breathe out for five seconds. You can count 1, 2, 3, 4, 5...1, 2, 3,

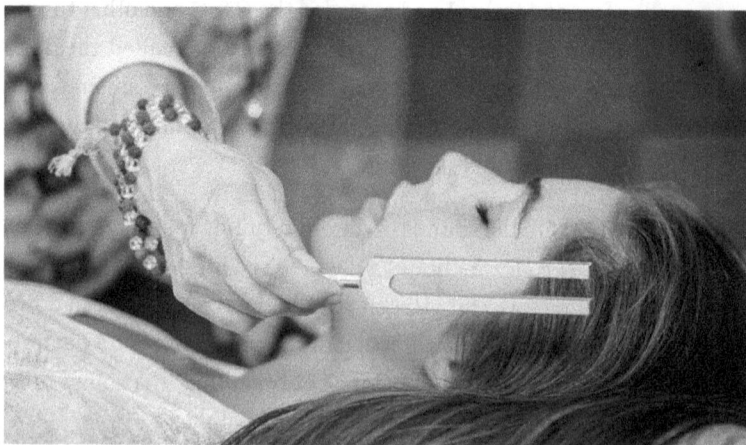

4, 5, and just get into that natural rhythm. I have seen that 5-second breathing is particularly effective for the generation of nitric oxide in the system. Breathing the right way, and mindful listening are both seen to be beneficial. The yogis of India discovered this many years ago, and then when we put these together in the modern context, they became even more effective. People do the Hatha yoga postures and combine them with the right breathing techniques, as well as the standalone breathing techniques called pranayama. So here, breathing and sound and movement go together and help to create that coherence within us.

I was doing this a lot whenever I went to Europe in the middle of the COVID pandemic and then the war. I saw such dismaying scenes at the airport. I was almost in tears, because I saw these people running around – stressed or troubled people who had no ability to self-regulate. So I would sit and just focus on my breath. I couldn't bring my tuning forks out in the airport, so I would just focus on breath and hum the sound of the C & G. I found that this practice worked really, really well.

The Vibrational Universe Decoded

While I have had excellent results while using, principally, the C and G tuning forks, the weighted 128 cycles per second fork is something else that I use and recommend. This type of fork has weights at the top, prongs, and then it has a stem, and I put a crystal on mine as well. The crystal isn't necessary, but it's nice. This works the same way as any tuning fork, but this has weights and is an octave lower. The weights cause more vibrations. So, when you tap it, say, on your knees or press it to your body, the weights cause it to shake a lot more. Therefore, you experience the vibration directly on your body a lot stronger. More than sound, it is the impact of the vibration on the body that actually goes to the same place as when it enters your ear. It's just a different pathway.

Tuning forks can be used on reflexology points, trigger points, and acupuncture points because this fits in with those systems perfectly. They can be used on different joints, or anywhere in the body. They can be used by anyone and are safe for most people: your family, kids, and friends.

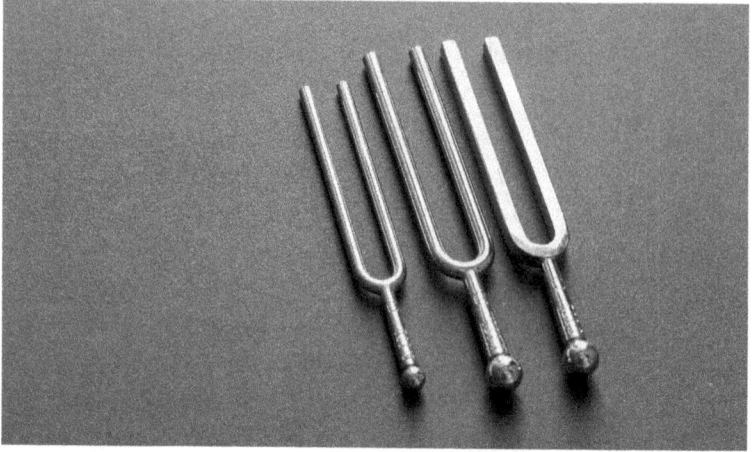

Qigong and tai chi are very integrated with these practices. You can move the body to the sound of the forks to help you. It helps with your regular meditative practice; to help you relax and feel better. I simply put them in my pocket and I carry them around. When I was in Europe working with Ukrainian refugees, I would just take these tuning forks and use them. I was amazed at the work I was able to do. Just three forks – you don't need much!

In recent times, COVID patients had been experiencing tinnitus, which is that constant ringing sound in the ear without any seeming stimuli. It may be possible to help such situations with sound healing. For instance, someone like a rock musician with exposure to very loud music experiencing tinnitus can respond quite effectively to sound therapy. As long as there is no structural issue, it is very possible to reverse the condition or mitigate it to a very large extent.

The thing to remember is that you mustn't put the fork on the head in the event of a concussion. Another warning is not to use it on the bones or joints of somebody with severe osteoporosis because this can cause the bones to crack.

Impact of Sound and Breathing on Your Health

To be clear, this isn't magic. It isn't something that you do one day and every health issue falls into place. This is a practice. It is an evolution and a process of refinement where each day you become better and your practice more effective. Like, say, psychotherapy, which takes many sessions – sometimes one step forward and a step back – to make progress. Again like psychotherapy, we integrate different practices and medical treatments to help and to become whole again. We work to create coherency and wholeness; sometimes we take the help of family and friends, whatever it takes to help us resolve things faster.

When you combine breathing and the sound therapy of the tuning forks in the optimal way, you will find an increase in the molecule nitric oxide. This is a gas manufactured in the neurons, the immune system, the lining of your blood vessels, and basically the circulatory system. And so the moment that this gas rises, it causes everything to relax; it triggers the relaxation response. Stress dissipates and everything lightens up. There is a continual pulse of the gas rising for three minutes, failing which the body experiences more stress and secretes more stress hormones. This in turn creates genetic breakdown, vascular breakdown, depression, body dysfunction, diabetes, motor neuron diseases, autoimmune diseases, and so on. These are all based fundamentally on the lack of this molecule in your body. So when you have a regular practice, you're encouraging your body to create this molecule every day naturally.

This is not to say that we can all be coherent all of the time, each day. This is impossible, just as it is impossible for an airplane to stay its course exactly 100% of the time. That is why self-regulation is so important. And that is what sound therapy can do for you. Along with the right breathing technique, it helps you self-regulate so that you can help your body create nitric oxide. Now I would urge people not to become dependent on the tuning forks. They're learning devices for your nervous system. You can and should be able to manage without them – by integrating breathing and mindfulness techniques. Consider how the yogis chant the sound OM as they intone certain mantras, or as some monastic orders make the humming sound, or the system of using sound bowls. All of these ancient systems came into being for some very good reasons.

Can Breathing Right Prolong Life?

There is some evidence to show that people who work in music live longer than the general population. Singers as well as music conductors appear to have longer lifespans, probably because of the sound and the vibrations that surround them for such significantly long periods. I myself am something of a sound hoarder, and I enjoy different sounds and frequencies. My studio is filled with different sounds such as from a piano, crystal bowls, and forks of various sorts. When I travel, my trusty forks are always in my suitcase, traveling right along with me: rugged, easily portable, and reliable.

It is simple to use these forks: simply tap them on the knee or on something a little hard and then hold them to the ears. Bring the fork up to the bone behind the ear to get the vibration going, and to let it spread out. You can also correspond to all the acupuncture points. In fact, I recommend combining sound therapy with integrative practices such as acupuncture, chiropractic osteopathic medicine, and so on.

Do this for a good minute or longer in the morning and then again at night. It is also a good idea to add this to active meditation practices, which is great to do at night, after a full day. It is like you become a conductor at night, conducting the sounds and moving with it. This helps you unwind and sleep better.

This is also an excellent accompaniment to Hatha yoga, tai chi, Qigong, and other practices. Whichever way works for you, however you can find time in a busy schedule, try to get attuned to your inner rhythms and find your coherence. This is something beyond the intellect; it is a body-mind experience.

When we are off-course we are likely to drift further and further off-course. However, if you have healthy practices in place, the mind, like a rubber band, will pull you back and keep you on course, bringing you back to your own center.

Those interested can visit my website for information on the protocols that can be used to combine tuning forks, breathwork, and other modalities to achieve healthy outcomes. For instance, the vagus protocol for the vagus nerve is something that I would recommend. The vagus nerve travels all the way from your head to your heart to your gut, and the vagus protocol shows you ways of working with that very simply. It adds a whole new dimension to using the tuning fork, because if there is one thing that really goes out of tune in the body, it is the vagus nerve more than anything else.

For those interested in sound healing, I would recommend my book, *Human Tuning: Sound Healing with Tuning Forks*, which answers your questions about sound healing, and integrates science, sound, and spirituality. My website, biosonics.com is a resource for sound healing products, Fibonacci brochure, music, photos, dance, articles and more. Readers will also find research papers covering topics such as:

• Sound Therapy Induced Relaxation: Down Regulating Stress Processes and Pathologies

• BioSonics, Stress Science, and Nitric oxide Literature Review

• Communication Between Animal Cells and the Plant Foods They Ingest: Phyto-Zooidal Dependencies and Signaling

• Tonal Nitric Oxide and Health: Anti-Bacterial and Viral Actions and Implications for HIV

• Cyclic Nitric Oxide Release by Human Granulocytes, and Invertebrate Ganglia and Immunocytes

• Nitric Oxide and Health

Now, at age 75, I consider myself retired from clinical practice. However, I still want to get the word out to as many people as possible about the efficacy of sound healing, how to use it in conjunction with breathing techniques and other therapeutic modalities. I also teach online and an in-person. I work with professionals and anyone who wants to learn sound healing. Being of assistance, and helping people heal and lead their best life is the most rewarding of experiences. I aim for simplicity, which is not easy for us – but when we achieve it, it works really well.

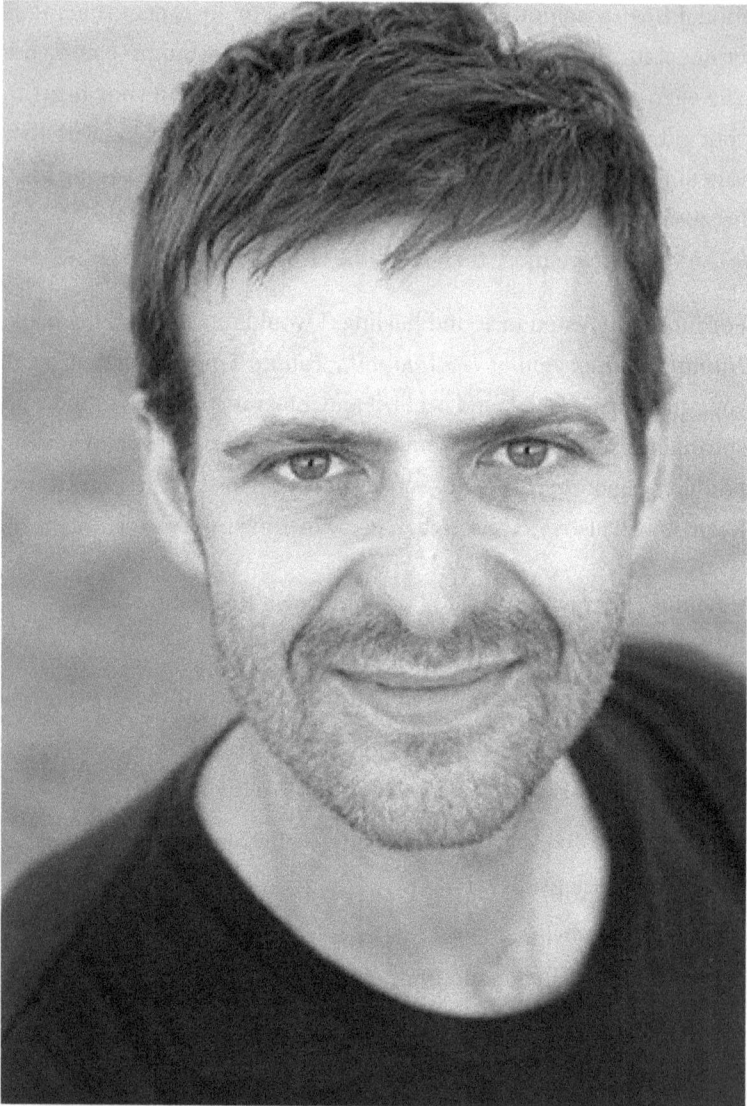

Jacob McGill

CHAPTER 7

BREATHING BIOMECHANICS: *Active respiration is a bit counterintuitive. Inhaling (breathing in) causes one set of intercostals to separate the ribs while the diaphragm contracts and pulls downward (creating a vacuum). Exhaling has two parts. The first is more of a release - the elasticity of the diaphragm's return moves upward to its dome shape. Contractions of the other breathing muscles can continue and can be used to push the last of the air out.*

HOW BREATHING HELPS WITH PAIN MANAGEMENT: BOTH CHRONIC & ACUTE

By Jacob McGill

I had my midlife crisis when I was 17. I was driving down a road that I had traveled my whole life. I was on the way home after school when I slid into a ditch after skidding on some gravel. I was going too fast. The truck somersaulted into the air, landed on the front, bounced up and down like a ball on a seal's nose, then landed on the roof. I was banged up and pretty near broken. The paramedics arrived and I was airlifted to the ICU. My veins had collapsed and they had to cut into my body to give me the IV. It was touch-and-go; I almost didn't make it. I have no memory of the event. I learned about it when I woke up from a coma in a hospital bed. I remained in the hospital for months, dealing with it all by using a lot of medication. There was excruciating pain, my mobility was significantly reduced, and I had yet to take the first step in what was to be a long journey of discovery, education, and healing.

I decided I wasn't going to settle for only being able to move my arm this high but not all the way. I decided I would not be content with limited mobility. I decided I would not live with the pain.

What I discovered about the human body, about pain, injury and healing, I now share with others. The Hundred Year Plan is what I use to help people with acute and chronic pain, musculoskeletal issues, degenerative issues, sciatica, arthritis, osteoporosis, back pain, posture problems, and more.

I help people become pain-free, avoid surgery, heal themselves, rebuild their strength, and increase mobility. I bring hope to people at a time when they feel they have to resign themselves to a restricted, limited life or the life of so-called "old age."

What I learned during the process of rehabilitation after my accident was an effective set of tools and a system of movement, meditation, conversations with the self, and yes, breathing. Learning how to breathe properly is a vital first step towards becoming pain-free.

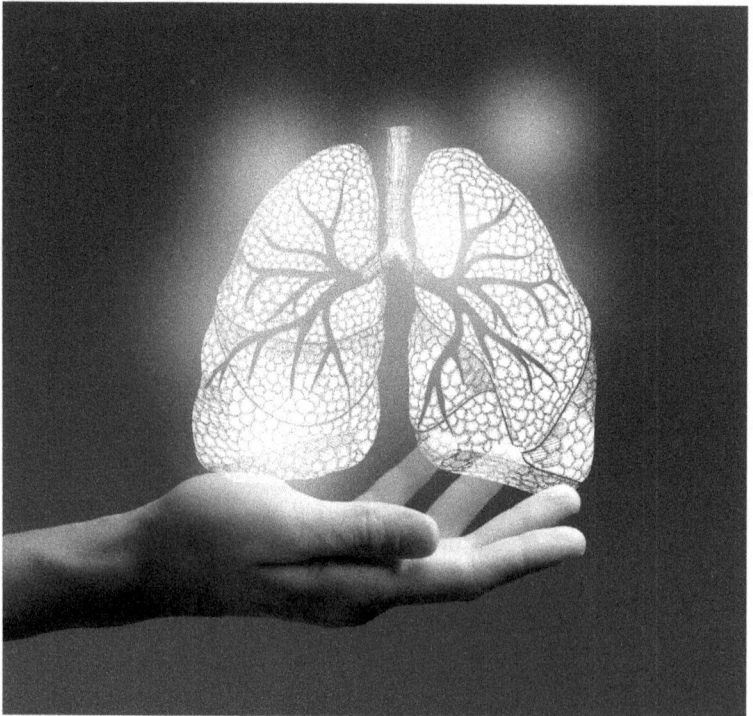

Are You Getting By on Fumes?

When we talk about being healthy, we always think about eating right, exercising, and hydrating. But most of us don't ever consider the one thing that we are doing 24x7 from the moment we are born – breathing. It is estimated that most people use just about 15% of their lung capacity.

Day-to-day most people aren't really breathing, they're just not dying. People are getting the mandatory minimum of respiration required to avoid a crisis. However, they aren't breathing the way they should.

When conscious breathing isn't practiced consistently, the body is basically getting by on fumes. Maybe the three days a week that somebody goes and exercises, or the two nights a week they go to yoga class might be the only time they breathe fully. Breathing consciously and correctly simply isn't a consistent part of everyday life for most people. If people are not breathing fully through the day, they are experiencing a net loss to their health, vitality, and well-being.

A significant portion of the population is breathing the wrong way and is unable to optimize the biomechanical aspects of breath, thus contributing to chronic pain, which is widespread. There is a shocking statistic that over 60% of the population over the age of 30 reports low back pain.

Shallow breathing, or breathing in the upper chest only, is disordered breathing. It's using about one-quarter of the available space. Incomplete inhalation and exhalation, yawning, breathlessness, fast breathing, and mouth breathing are some symptoms of disordered breathing. This impacts the autonomic nervous system, which in turn affects immunity, fertility, digestion, and growth. Noticeably, this can cause brain fog, anxiety, dizziness, pins and needles, even pain, and lead to feeling overwhelmed.

Devoting just 30 minutes a week to breathing the right way can help optimize performance and well-being. I have been taught breathing techniques for martial arts, meditation, rehabilitation, and performance athletics use, and found them effective for managing pain and improving well-being.

Applying the appropriate method can help change the body's chemistry, and create new and supportive states to impact nervous system responses, improve posture, and promote better physical health. If you have ever studied movement, someone probably told you how posture is central to structural health. And breath and posture are intrinsically connected.

Understanding the Biomechanics Of Breathing

The biomechanics of breathing are important to understand. There are 21 breathing or respiratory muscles, 20 of which are postural muscles. Relative to breathing, only the diaphragm isn't a postural muscle. So, it is easy to see how improving posture helps us breathe better and vice versa. Researchers have found that poor posture can contribute to gastrointestinal pain, lower back pain, neck pain, and even muscle weakness in some areas - and breath is intrinsic to posture.

The diaphragm stands at the core of respiration. It is also responsible for hiccupping, coughing, laughing, sighing, and so on. These are recovery breaths, or somatic-type of breaths that take place unconsciously. Other muscles are involved but the diaphragm is vitally important. It contracts to push air out during the exhale, then snaps back to create a vacuum and pulls air back into the lungs.

The body learns through movement, so I believe the best way to improve breathing is to connect it to movement. This can be total body movement or something more rehab-based where a portion of the body is stabilized while another area "works out."

Moving this way can teach the body to breathe in the "right relationship" to the activity. For example, our shoulder blades spread apart instinctively during an inhalation, so deliberately moving the arms apart matched with an exhalation and together with an inhalation is natural.

Of course, the ideal inhalation and exhalation is 360 degrees. It involves all 21 respiratory muscles and moves the ribs and the vertebrae, the physics of the musculoskeletal /respiratory system.

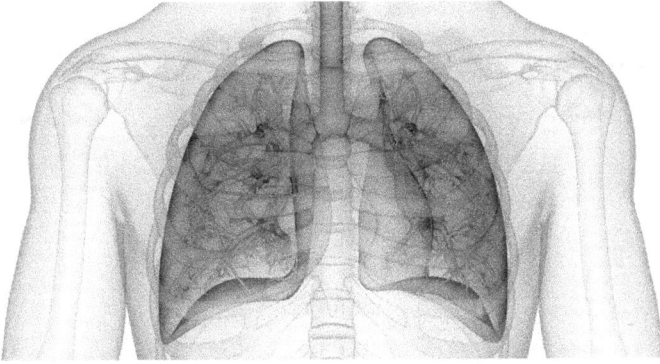

Relax Your Way into Better Mental Focus

The physical action of breathing impacts almost everything in the body. For instance, behind the lungs are the 12 thoracic vertebrae, and attached to each of those vertebrae are the ribs. In a sense, every breath is an opportunity to compress and decompress the spine, and to move around the cerebrospinal fluid, which enables the brain and body to function much better.

Breathing also helps massage the organs above and below the diaphragm as well as what passes through it including the aorta, esophagus and vagus nerve. As long as the supporting (core) musculature is healthy and balanced, i.e. the body is active and fit, the right breathing techniques can be tremendously beneficial.

Changing how you breathe can help improve circulation and delivery of oxygen to and removal of carbon dioxide from the vital systems of the body, enhance structural well-being, and improve immunity. It can also improve focus and acuity while helping the body relax and relieve symptoms of anxiety and depression. The mind becomes calmer, and is better equipped to handle stress. This will also help to improve quality of sleep since all of these systems are closely interlinked. If someone has frequent headaches, chronic pain, fatigue, sleep issues, or brain fog, it is quite possible to create some relief by improving breathing.

Additionally, there is the psychological aspect of breathing. Most of us have seen how the simple action of taking deep, regular breaths in a stressful situation helps us calm down. We feel more in control,

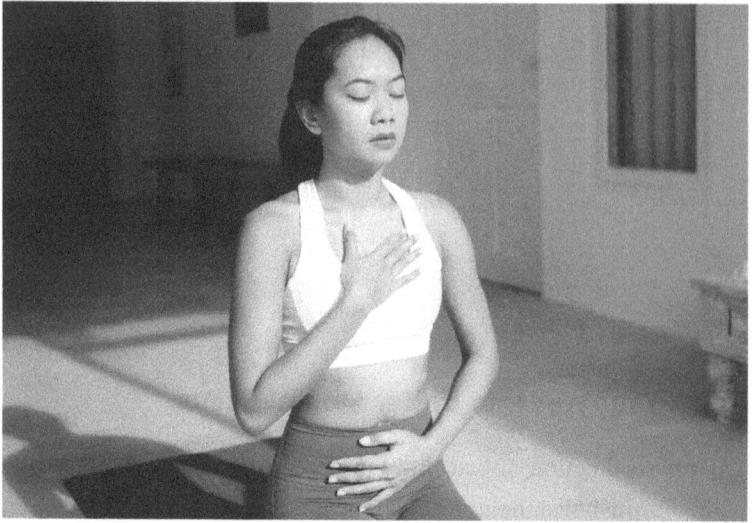

our mind is clearer, and we give ourselves the time to make better decisions – the chance to be fully alive in the moment. There is a reason why Olympic athletes spend time visualizing their events. It helps to engage the system in different ways and makes the mind a partner in the process.

Deliberate breathing can also help regulate the flow of energy in the body – all reasons why it can help us perform better physically, mentally, and emotionally.

The Power of Back Breathing

When I first learned about back breathing, it was an enlightening experience. Typically, we are a little dissociated from our bodies, but breathing into the back makes us breathe intentionally, conscious of the body, the back, and all the muscles involved in the process. A considerable volume of the lungs sits behind our midline and that's the space we could be breathing into. We need to target those muscles intentionally, like putting air between our shoulder blades. This is a part of the rehabilitation process that helps bring people back to health and restores function. By focusing on the duration, the frequency, and the range of motion of breathing, we can rebuild the benefit. We want to create healthy habits – consciously and deliberately.

An important aspect of my rehabilitation process after my accident was Pilates, which emphasizes specific breathing techniques paired with movement. The penultimate Pilates exercise is called The Hundreds: traditionally, you breathe in five times through the nose and then out five times through the mouth.

The first goal point is to establish a pattern of the breath - consciously inhaling reps and then exhaling reps - to reinforce the brain-body connection while firing specific muscles. Kind of like doing biceps and then triceps during a workout.

After practicing this a few times, the second aspect pays attention to volume. You start with the four inhales and use the fifth to fill the lungs completely. Repeat with the exhales: four out and then absolutely empty. This helps the Brain/Body map the volume we normally don't use; it accesses the areas of the lungs and the range of motion of our breathing muscles we often neglect. For example, we have two sets of intercostal muscles (muscles right between the ribs). One set pulls the ribs apart (to inhale) and the other pulls them together (to exhale). The reps of The Hundreds stretch and strengthen both directly, while recruiting other breathing muscles. There are a lot of traditional breathing techniques, also now supported by the current research, that point to the importance not just of inhaling but also of exhaling through the nose. (While this is true, Pilates Breathing created by Joseph Pilates requires exhalation via the mouth.) Nose exhalation has a specific application and purpose. The forced exhale, recruiting all 21 breathing muscles while actively using the abdominals and core, is a fundamental part of the Pilates work. The "Oral Exhale" is there for a reason – a full and complete exhalation with contraction. Pilates said "You have to out the air to in the air."

The Eternal Exhale. Letting Go of It All

The important thing is communicating with the nervous system. Each person will have a different way. When I'm helping someone overcome pain, we sift through the clutter of information that typically surrounds us. We work to become adept at listening to the body, and to progress in natural and safe ways.

Another breathing technique is something I call the "Eternal Exhale." This is the diaphragmatic reset. It is a part of the yawning function that engages a shunt point in the lungs. Usually, even when we exhale, we don't really empty our lungs. This technique is about a gradual process as though we were trying to exhale forever. The body wants to inhale. We want to learn to ignore the instinct. It's kind of like holding your breath but on the exhale. The exercise is to exhale, exhale, exhale, pause and feel the urge to inhale, then exhale a couple more times. In a sense, you want to lean into the seeming discomfort. The goal of the practice is to allow the elasticity of all your tissue to take over – a little like the wringing of a wet towel.

There are other breathing techniques such as expelling breath in a way that allows a person to go deeper into water. Then there is the 4-7-8 technique (which goes as far back as the teachings of Patanjali) that is useful for calming the nervous system.

I believe the most important skill is to learn to listen to the body rather than being pedantic about any exercise. One of my primary goals when working with clients is to help them learn to listen to their bodies. I'm like a marriage counselor between the client and their proprioceptive nervous system. I help them understand what the body is saying and get them to a point where the communication is so effective that I am no longer needed. It is this learning – developing the ability to listen to the body – that supports longevity and freedom.

Breathing Through Pain Relief

It is my aim to help people enter a pathway to resolving pain through the body or the mind. Some breathing techniques have been around for centuries, such as the ones from the Yoga Sutras. While they can work well for some, they may not for someone who is in a lot of pain, someone who cannot fill their lungs completely. A lot of the pranayama techniques require forceful or vigorous breathing that can be both uncomfortable and contraindicated. So, people in a lot of pain can start with small breaths, doing what they can without stressing out while paying attention to themselves and following the pathway. The nervous system is highly intelligent and gives us a lot of freedom! Gradually, the body builds capacity, and the breathing works in tandem with other modalities to help reduce pain.

Listen to Your Body; It Tells You a Lot

Talking about learning to listen to the body reminds me of a French Canadian guy who ran an office where I worked one summer during college. He was a smoker and generally a vegetarian. He told me that when he went shopping, he would smell the items and whatever smelled good to him is what went in his basket. He said that sometimes he would be out and cooking meat smelled good, and when it did he'd get some and eat it. He told me that it would taste good at first and he would eat until "the taste changed" and then he would stop.

He fed his body based on smell – a clever way of bridging the sympathetic to the parasympathetic nervous systems. This is just one example of listening to what the body says, wants, and needs.

My grandmothers were great examples. Both lived through World War II and suffered significant hardships. They also both passed on at about the same age in their mid-80s. However, there was a world of difference in their quality of life. One decayed in a hospital bed with a body that had been falling apart for years. (I noticed her posture degrading when I was 10.) My other grandmother outlived her third husband. When she was moved to a place without a garden, she marched over to my aunt's, ripped up the yard, and planted one. This is a great example of how our mindset impacts our lives, our health, and well-being. My grandmother wasn't saving the oceans or leading people, but she had an attitude that said, I'm busy; I've got stuff to do. Her outlook gave her a certain aspect of longevity – not just lifespan but healthspan.

For us to improve our healthspan for the duration of our lifespan, proper breathing is vital and fundamental. It isn't very difficult. It does not require a lot of effort. All we have to do is apply some conscious thought and consistent practice. Maybe you won't notice any big changes right away. However, the internal changes that the right breathing techniques bring about will help you create vitality now and remain well into your later years.

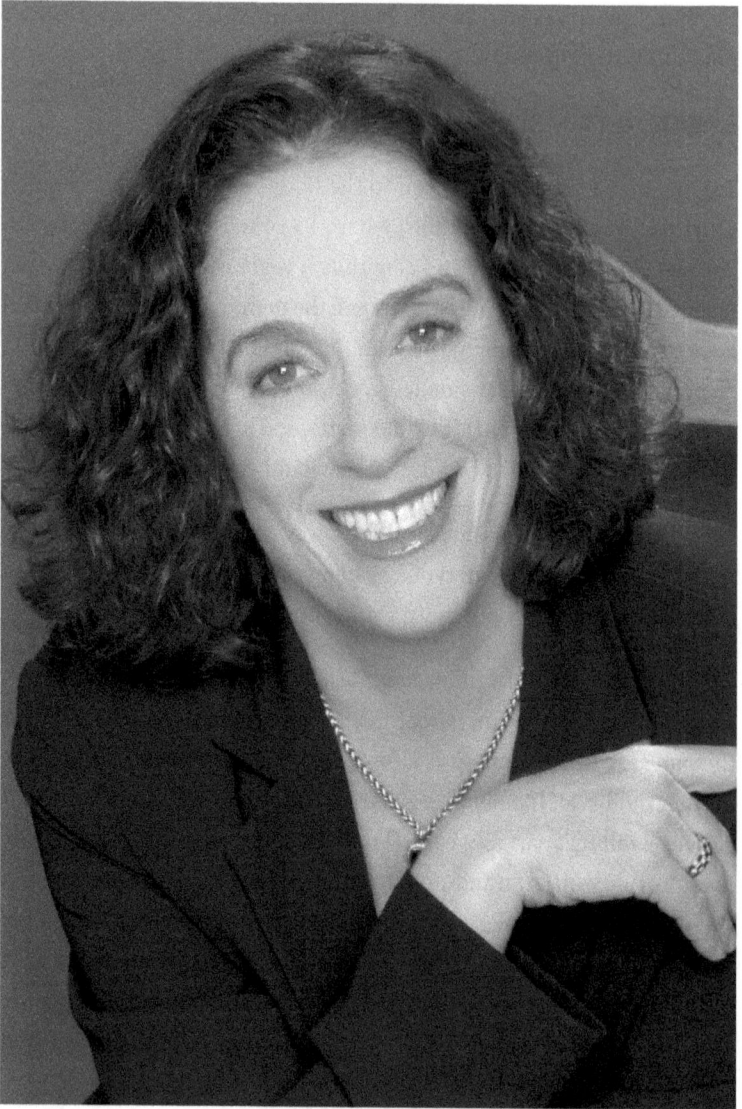

Anat Baniel

CHAPTER 8

*Your brain is the "CEO" of all that you do. **NeuroMovement**® is a novel approach that communicates with the brain through movement and 9 Essentials. It upgrades thequality of the functioning of the brain itself, and thus transforms the field of possibilities, going beyond what you might otherwise believe to be possible.*

*There is no one "right" or "correct" way to breathe. There are many ways to breathe well. The "boss" of your breathing, and all movements that you do, is your brain! With **NeuroMovement**® you can activate your brain to learn how to engage your back, ribs, sternum, pelvis, diaphragm, and your whole body to spontaneously breathe better and feel better in new and exciting ways.*

NEUROMOVEMENT®: IMPROVE YOUR BREATHING THROUGH POSITIVE BRAIN CHANGE

By Anat Baniel & Dr. Neil Sharp

We've known for millennia that breathing is central to life and the quality with which we breathe influences everything in us, including our moods, thinking, well-being, stamina, and health. The quality of our breathing can vary tremendously from limited and challenged due to disease, psychological issues, environmental stressors, and poor habits, to wonderfully free, vibrant, and empowering. The big question is, is there a way that we can intentionally improve the way we breathe, and if so, then how?

The answer is a definite yes. There are many approaches to help enhance the quality of our breathing and that's what our *NeuroMovement*®: *Breathing for Life* course is all about.

There are four main points we focus on through the course:

- Becoming free of the notion that there is the right way to breathe and discovering different ways to breathe that give us greater freedom and potency in breathing, body, and mind.

- Breathing is an automatic function, not a voluntary one. We can control our breath for short periods of time because the muscles that are involved in breathing, aside from the diaphragm itself, are under our voluntary control. This creates the opportunity for us to expand the freedom and dexterity with which we use these muscles that in turn will *spontaneously* improve the way we breathe.

- What regulates and controls the way we breathe and the *quality* with which we breathe, is the brain. The brain organizes our movement, and movement is at the heart of breathing. How we move, and how the different parts of our body dynamically relate to each other as we breathe, will decide the quality of our breath. When we want to change and improve the way we breathe, we need to change what the brain "tells" the body to do.

- The brain can, and does, change itself throughout life. For *positive* brain change to happen, the brain needs new information. The main source of such information for the brain is movement coupled with attention, slowing down, reduction of force, imagination, awareness, and lots of variability. (Six of what I call The *Nine Essentials of NeuroMovement*®)

Movement is the main driver of the creation of new neural connections, what is often referred to as brain mapping. When new connections and new neural networks are created in the brain, the ability to spontaneously breathe better emerges.

The How

One of the characteristics of healthy breathing is that it changes spontaneously to meet the demands of the moment. When we run fast to catch a bus, in no time we breathe very differently than when we are sitting on a sofa watching a fun TV show. That means that we need to

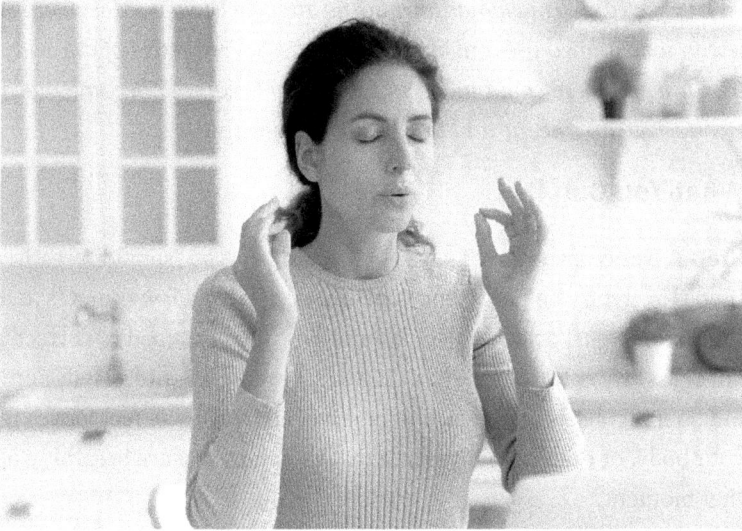

have a wide variety of ways to breathe available to us. The sedentary lifestyle that so many of us live, combined with a limited movement repertoire that is deeply habituated, leads to reduced capacity and vibrancy in our breathing.

The good news is that the brain is always ready to change, learn, and improve on itself when given a chance. This is true for young, or old, healthy, or those suffering from conditions that interfere with breathing.

Years ago, I worked with a lovely 12-year-old girl, Samantha, who had severe scoliosis. (Scoliosis is a sideways curvature of the spine that can vary in its severity.) Normally, severe scoliosis has negative impact on breathing. In addition to back pain and hoping to avoid surgery, Samantha really wanted to take ballet lessons. She could not do so because her breathing, and stamina, were too diminished by her condition. After working together for a few months, the curvature decreased some, even though it was still significant. However, through the process Samantha's brain learned more differentiated, refined, intricate, and complex ways to organize her movements so that her breathing got freer and fuller to the point that she was able to join ballet classes and do everything that the other girls did, do it well, and for extended periods of time.

In her words: *"The change during and after each (NeuroMovement®) lesson was immediate and enormous. I discovered parts of my body that I never knew could move so freely. My breathing became much steadier as my ribcage and chest learned to be free."*

What You Can Do:

Step 1: Notice if you have an idea or ideas of how you "should" breathe. If you do, gently begin freeing yourself, even if for a few minutes at a time, from your, or other people's notions of what "good", "correct", or "right" ways to breathe are. Instead become an interested, non-judgmental observer of how you breathe, and what you feel moves in your body, or does not move, that results in how you are breathing at that moment.

Step 2: Many of us, at least some of the time, tend to have disordered breathing patterns due to anxiety or stress. The body's natural response to fear and anxiety is a form of freezing and limiting our mobility. The belly gets pulled in and held in, the movement of the sternum, the ribs, and the spine gets restricted.

For breathing to occur air needs to be sucked into the lungs and expelled out of the lungs. Fundamentally this is done by expanding and contracting the volume of the chest cavity. This can be done in many ways, but gets hugely diminished when movement of the chest, pelvis, shoulders, shoulder blades, sternum, and spine are limited.

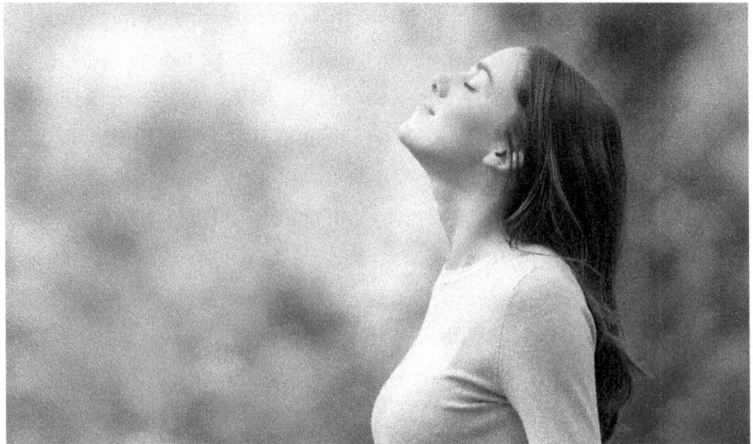

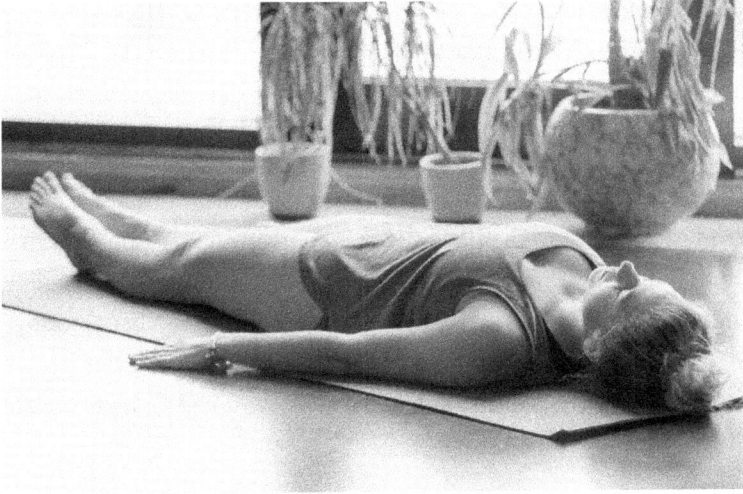

Imagine that your spine, ribs in the back, sides, and front, and the sternum, clavicles, shoulder blades, and diaphragm *create a box*. Imagine this box to have very flexible corners and sides. Begin doing simple movements, either in sitting, standing, or lying down and feel/imagine what happens to the shape of the "box" as you move. For example, in sitting, begin turning slowly right and left, and feel how the "box" changes it shape. *Reduce the effort* in which you do the movement and let the "box" change its shape more and more as you twist from side to side. Be sure to move slowly, *keep reducing the effort* with which you do the movement, and *move only in the range that feels comfortable*. After 3-5 minutes of doing this movement, stop, sit quietly, and simply let the breath form itself. Notice if it has become easier, lighter, fuller, with less effort, or not. Notice if your general feeling of self has changed, and in what ways.

You can then repeat the same twisting movement and imagining the box in other positions such as lying, bending down, standing etc.

Step 3: Most people move in ways that are poorly organized mechanically and neurologically. These ways of moving become habitual. That means that most people habitually move with too much effort and insufficient differentiation of their movements. A very common response when trying to perform a movement is to push harder, try to stretch the muscles, and go too fast so it is hard to be aware of what one is doing. Beyond looking to improve the performance of any specific movement, including breathing, in step 3 we invite you to begin paying attention to the HOW, the underlying way in which you do any movement.

What we propose is that when you want to learn a new movement, or improve on movements that you are already doing, you shift to a more "mindful" way. To improve any movement that we do, including breathing, the exact opposite of the usual way most people move is needed. Instead of pushing, rushing, forcing, ignoring pain and discomfort, and being unaware of what we are doing and how we are doing it, we intentionally:

- slow down the movements – fast we can only do what we already know

- reduce the force with which we do the movements – the greater the force the less we feel what we do and the brain has no new information to work with

- look away from trying to reach our goals at that moment – make space for the new, i.e. learning, to occur

- and shift our attention to what we feel as we move to guide us.

Take a few minutes every so often in your exercise routine, or in any of your daily movements, and intentionally do them smaller, slower, with as little force as you can muster, so you can become aware of what you are doing and what you feel as you move. See if in those few minutes you can bring the movements that you are doing to the point of comfort and safety. After 4-5 minutes, stop, be still, and feel and observe how you feel and how you breathe.

Step 4: Often when people try to improve their breathing, they try to inhale as much air as they can. Once again, the opposite is what is needed. One of the fastest and surest ways to improve breathing is to focus on the exhalation. Moshé Feldenkrais and Carl Stough, both of whom I was fortunate to study with, understood that the longer and fuller the exhalation, the better we will breathe without trying.

To experience this for yourself, lie on your back, take a brief inhalation, then begin counting gently out loud, at a good speed, perhaps one number per second, or a bit faster, as long as you can maintain the same speed, until you run out of air. Then wait for the air to be passively sucked in and again exhale as slowly and gently, and as long as you can, and allow the air to come in when it is done as if by itself. Do this for 2-3 minutes. Then do the same in two or three additional positions such as lying on your side, then standing on all fours, sitting in a chair etc. In each new position do the above described for 2-3 minutes. Feel how when you change positions and do the movements as recommended above, the breathing changes. When you are done with at least 3 positions, lie on your back and once again count as you exhale and notice if your exhale is longer. Then simply lie quietly and notice how you feel in general and how your breathing forms itself now.

Changing the Brain and Improving Breathing One Movement at a Time

The brain's power to change is really quite remarkable, which is what we look to harness with Anat Baniel Method® NeuroMovement®. It is the work we do to wake up the brain to create new connections and new patterns, and with it new possibilities. Breathing for Life is a NeuroMovement® program, which I have developed in collaboration with Pete Bissonnette, CEO of Learning Strategies. It consists of 10 NeuroMovement® lessons designed to improve breathing, movement, and awareness skills. It also includes an introduction by Dr. Neil Sharp, a former physician and professional opera singer, as well as a 45-minute Q&A session with me.

Some of the outcomes reported by those who participated in the *Breathing for Life NeuroMovement®* are increased energy and stamina, improved resilience, feeling calmer, sleeping better, reduced pain, and clearer thinking. People who have done this program also report increased general mobility, as well as greater awareness of the rib cage, spine, clavicles, sternum, diaphragm, and other areas involved in breathing.

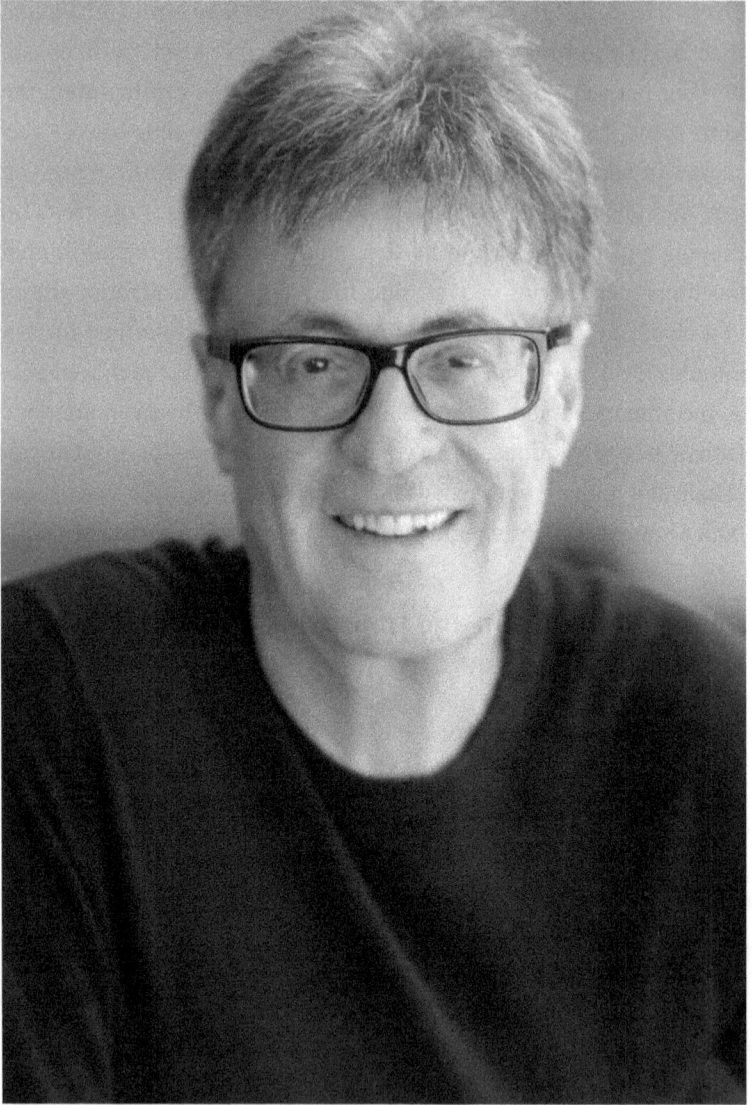

Adiel Gorel

CLOSING STATEMENT

IN CLOSING

By Adiel Gorel

Every expert who wrote a chapter in this book inspired me, and it is my great hope that they have inspired you as well.

I greatly enjoyed each and every interview, and felt gratified I could ask and delve deep into points I wasn't clear about.

Sometimes, in these busy times, we don't necessarily have the time to read an entire book that may reflect the life-long work or study of the author. For me, having this book available as a resource is gratifying. The fact that each of the experts took the time to distill their knowledge into a single chapter enables me, and I hope you, to read the essence of their work in a concentrated form. Having this on my bookshelf, ready to quickly remind myself of the subject of each chapter, feels like I have a useful resource.

Having read the book, I once again was reminded of the myriad ways we can improve our life just by doing simple, achievable things, which cost very little or nothing at all. I can see our daily habits can be reset to serve our health, or can easily slide into a default that we set long ago, perhaps even unconsciously, that could be hindering our vitality.

Reflecting, with gratitude, on what I learned from this book, I hope you find the information usable and easy to apply in ways that improve your vitality and enjoyment.

Dr. Nathan Bryan goes to the heart of the matter: he talks about the multiple benefits of nitric oxide. Much of what we accomplish via correct breathing, humming, and other techniques, may just boil down to increasing our supply of nitric oxide. Nathan reminds us of the simple changes we can make to increase that supply. He talks about eating dark green leafy vegetables, humming, chewing our food very well, and not destroying our beneficial bacteria in the mouth cavity. His advice is accessible, doable, and affordable. I find that exciting, as I know that the more we complicate things, the less likely we will implement them in our daily lives. Simplicity is exciting, isn't it? Especially when it comes to improving our health.

Patrick McKeown talks to us about the importance of breathing through the nose as well. He talks about gentle breath holding to build carbon dioxide. He emphasizes the BOLT (Breath Oxygen Level Test) score, and how a higher BOLT score correlates with overall better health. The BOLT score can be gradually improved. Everything Patrick suggests can be implemented easily and at hardly any cost.

Andi and Jonathan Goldman dive deeper into the benefits of humming. Others have already talked about how we generate much more nitric oxide when we hum. Andi and Jonathan refine humming, and, besides the obvious benefits, show us we can direct the energy of the hum into healing parts of our body. They connect humming back to the ancient practice in Southeast Asia, and remind us, once again, how something so simple and easy, which costs nothing, can improve our lives. We can hum in the car, at home, and while walking. Everywhere. Are you humming right now? I am as I write this for you. It's simple and fun and healthy.

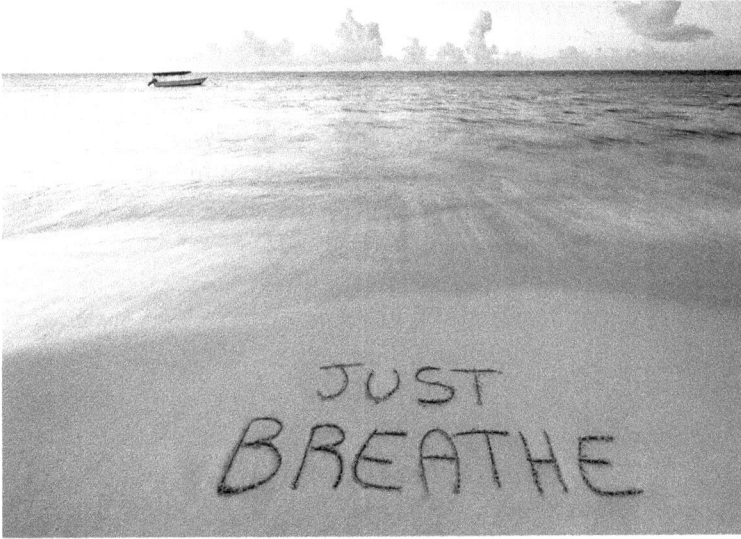

Even if we breathe efficiently, we could be inhaling damaging materials and bringing them into our bodies. Beth Greer made us aware of the toxins and pollutants we could be breathing in our own home: VOCs, chemicals from fragrances, dust and mold particles, and many other elements that we can bring into our body by breathing them in. Beth gave us practical advice as to how to minimize these harmful particles in our home. Simple, wonderful solutions that benefit our whole family.

Dr. Erlene Chiang talked about the Yin and Yang aspects of our existence, about breathing and Qi, and about the benefits that Qigong and tai chi can have on our health in general, and our breathing in particular. She talks about restoring balance, breathing with the total capacity of our lungs, and living in harmony with the natural cycles.

Anat Baniel talked about attaining better freedom of movement in our body, by variations of movements that show our brain we can move our chest, shoulders, and sternum in ways that are freer than our habitual norm. Moving freely creates more space for our lungs to expand, and may allow the diaphragm to move better, thus improving our breathing. Having worked with Anat, I can attest, from personal experience, to the joy of moving and breathing more freely after a movement lesson by Anat.

Jacob McGill talked about breathing as part of the whole of the movement of our body. He discussed "back breathing" and how it enables us to get more air into the lungs. He discussed various breathing exercises, such as the "Eternal Exhale," and the ancient "4-7-8" breathing. He also talked about breathing as an integral part of dealing with and healing pain.

James Nestor talked to us about breathing through the nose, and the intricate and specialized network we have behind our nose made explicitly for breathing. I actually started taping my mouth at night, so as to make sure I breathe through my nose, years before. I was inspired by Patrick McKeown's first book *Close Your Mouth*. I loved how James Nestor shared the story of the measurements taken at the Stanford Sleep Lab. He and his associate had their noses plugged up, and for ten days they were made to only breathe through their mouths. Multiple measurements were taken. Then the process was reversed: their mouths were taped for ten days, so they breathed only through the nose. Extensive measurements were taken at the sleep lab. The difference was enormous. The improvement achieved by simply nose breathing was remarkable. James talks about the production of nitric oxide, and how we produce much more nitric oxide when we breathe through our nose. We produce even more when we hum. The notion of nitric oxide production via nose breathing and humming keeps repeating itself throughout the book, coming from different experts.

James also talks about the importance of chewing, and how in modern life we chew much less than we used to in the past. He recommends chewing more, and some chewing gums that he finds useful. Everything he shared, which can make such a huge difference in our lives, is either free or quite inexpensive, and does not require much time. James was interviewed by me on *The Adiel Gorel Show*, but due to publishing rights, his chapter was not included in the book. Nevertheless, you can access the interview on all podcast channels, like YouTube, Spotify, Apple Podcast, etc. Just look for *The Adiel Gorel Show* and the James Nestor Interview.

I talked to a friend of mine, an MD. I shared what I had learned about nose breathing, but his opinion was that "air is air and it doesn't matter how you breathe it in." It is gratifying to see that slowly, even medical professionals are starting to realize the benefits of nose breathing. The measurements at the Stanford Sleep Lab should be enough to win over any skeptical MD.

John Beaulieu highlights how simple it is to use basic sounds made by simple tuning forks to regulate ourselves, and heal injury via touching the weighted fork to our body. He mentions humming and the profound effect it can have for us. He talks about a very simple 5-breath and the results he saw it has on people, including himself. Reading about how the anechoic chamber presented him with the auditory results of what happens when he is upset and anxious is revealing: how many hours and days do we walk around in that state? What if we could quickly mitigate it with humming or a couple of tuning forks used for just a few minutes? He also gets back to what virtually every expert on breathing touches upon – nitric oxide and its production. It's inspiring to me that John's methods are so simple, accessible, and either free or inexpensive. Everyone could benefit from applying them to daily life, especially since it also takes little time to do.

Every one of the experts featured in this book ultimately harks back to breathing naturally, using the full capacity of our lungs. They talk about breathing through our nose as an important factor. We create the precious nitric oxide gas more when we breathe through our noses, and when we hum. As I delighted in mentioning many times before, I am gratified that very simple actions, with no need for much time or financial investment, and with little effort, can yield positive differences in the most fundamental bodily function. I sincerely hope that this book has been, and will be, useful and beneficial to you, the reader. I hope you employ the simple-to-follow advice given by the experts who wrote it, and that you feel inspired to go deeper into what they teach, and gain mastery in improving your breathing and your life.

ABOUT THE AUTHORS

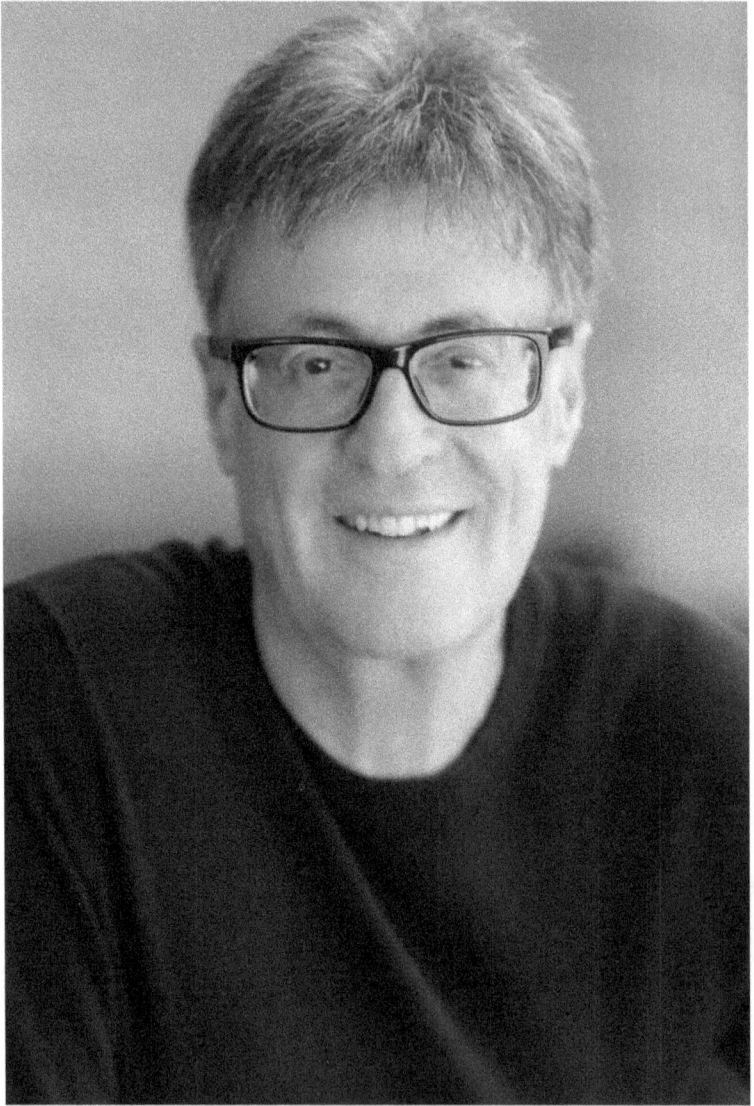

Adiel Gorel

Adiel Gorel

Adiel Gorel is the CEO of a San Francisco Bay Area real estate investment firm, and has helped thousands achieve their long-term financial goals. Adiel wears many hats, one of which is that of a passionate health seeker looking to bring about positive change using natural, intuitive methods. Adiel has been fascinated by the idea of breathing the right way; by the idea that we can all breathe our way to good health. Over the years, he has read various books, studied the methods used by different breathing experts, and been a committed proponent of nasal breathing. *The Adiel Gorel Show* is one of the ways in which he strives to get out the message of healthy breathing habits to his listeners, hoping to drive change via this simple lifestyle change. This book is a labor of love – a collection of essays from breathing experts; people from different walks of life who share their experiences, techniques, and unique insights into breathing.

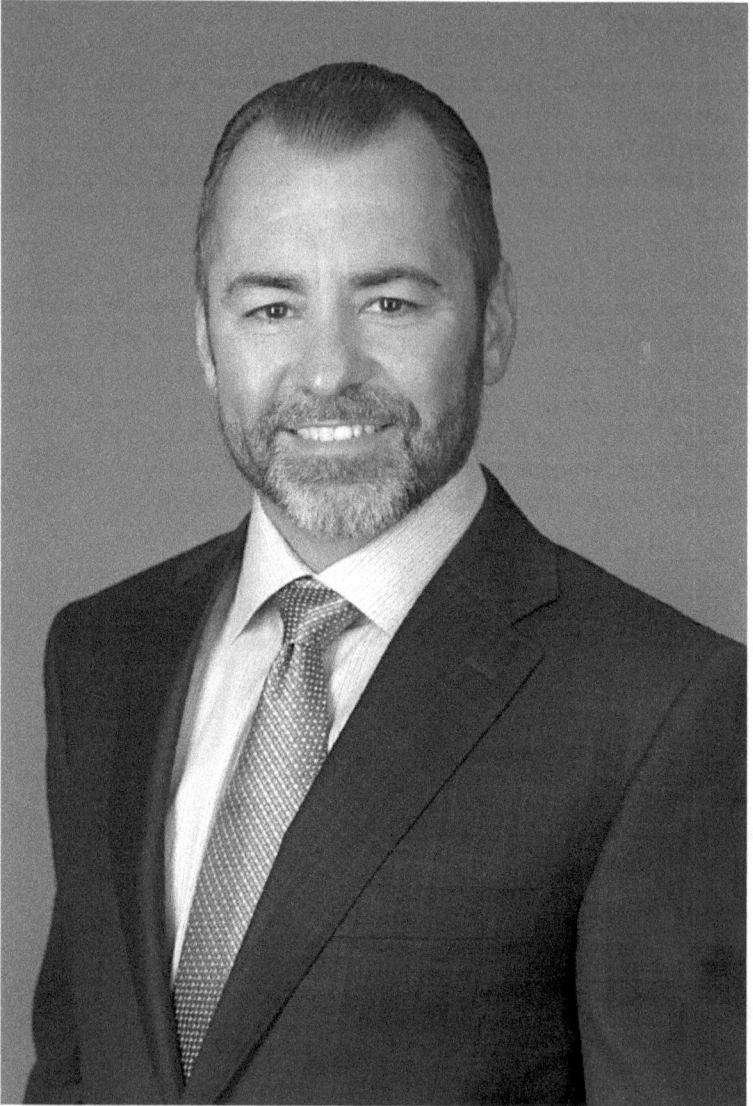

Dr. Nathan S. Bryan

Dr. Nathan Bryan

Dr. Bryan earned his undergraduate Bachelor of Science degree in Biochemistry from the University of Texas at Austin, and his doctoral degree from Louisiana State University School of Medicine in Shreveport where he was the recipient of the Dean's Award for Excellence in Research. He pursued his post-doctoral training as a Kirschstein Fellow at Boston University School of Medicine in the Whitaker Cardiovascular Institute. After a two-year post-doctoral fellowship, in 2006 Dr. Bryan was recruited to join faculty at the University of Texas Health Science Center at Houston by Ferid Murad, M.D., Ph.D., 1998 Nobel Laureate in Medicine or Physiology. Dr. Bryan has been involved in nitric oxide research for the past 20 years and has made many seminal discoveries in the field. His many seminal discoveries have resulted in dozens of issued US and International patents, and the product technology resulting from his discoveries and inventions has improved patient care worldwide. Dr. Bryan is a successful entrepreneur and Founder of HumanN, Inc, Pneuma Nitric Oxide, LLC., Nitric Oxide Innovations, LLC and Bryan Nitriceuticals, LLC. His product technology is responsible for hundreds of millions of product sales worldwide. Most recently, Dr. Bryan serves as Founder and CEO of Nitric Oxide Innovations, LLC, a privately-held, clinical-stage biopharmaceutical company that is actively engaged in the discovery and development of nitric oxide based therapies. Their lead drug candidate, NOviricid, is currently in phase 3 clinical trials for the treatment of COVID19 in African Americans and Hispanics. Dr. Bryan is an international leader in molecular medicine and nitric oxide biochemistry.

As such, Dr. Bryan has also been working to produce useful products that deliver nitric oxide effectively, such as mouth dissolving lozenges that were launched successfully some years ago. NO Beetz is a recently launched product, a beet extract powder that helps deliver this molecule safely and effectively to users.

NO2U.com
N101.com
nitricoxideinnovations.com

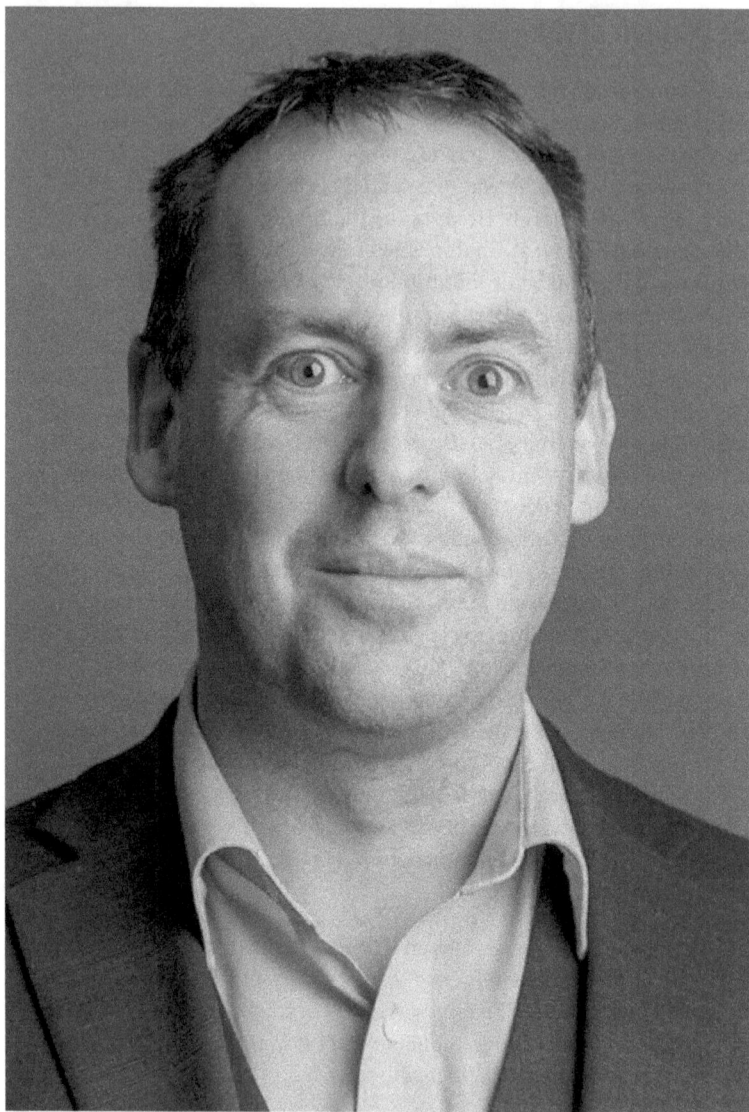

Patrick McKeown

Patrick McKeown

Patrick McKeown is the creator, CEO, and Director of Education and Training at Oxygen Advantage®, Director of Education and Training at Buteyko Clinic International, and President of Buteyko Professionals International. He is a leading international expert on breathing and sleep, and the author of bestselling books including *The Oxygen Advantage*.

The Oxygen Advantage® is a unique breath-work training program developed by him, focusing on helping people breathe better, feel better, and achieve their potential. People receive training to breathe the right way. They become fitter and stronger, reduce breathlessness, and relieve the symptoms of many common illnesses. They experience increased exercise intensity with less effort, and improved energy levels, concentration, and mental focus. The program includes simulating high altitude training to improve aerobic and anaerobic capacity.

Patrick recommends many products: The purpose-built nasal dilator to help athletes achieve optimal sports breathing, The Oxygen Advantage® sports mask for new levels of fitness and performance, and MYOTAPE, a lip tape for habitual mouth breathers that helps them reduce snoring, symptoms of asthma, and improves sleep quality. Patrick McKeown is also the author of the 2021 bestselling book *The Breathing Cure: Habits for a Healthier, Happier and Longer Life*, which consists of self-practice breathing exercises for people of all ages.

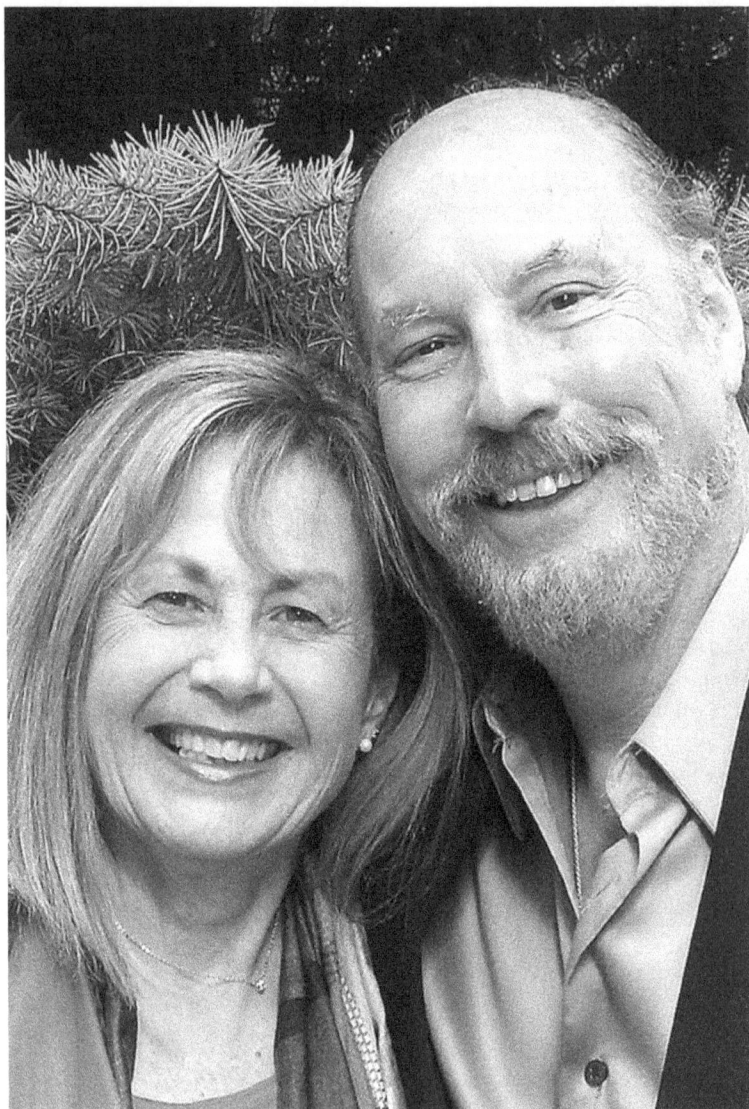

Andi & Jonathan Goldman

Andi & Jonathan Goldman

Jonathan Goldman is a leading expert in sound healing and harmonics. He has worked with sound in scientific and spiritual traditions. He is empowered by the Chant Master of the Dalai Lama's Drepung Loseling Monastery to teach Tibetan Overtone Chanting. His collaborative work "Tibetan Master Chants" was nominated for a 2006 Grammy Award for "Best Traditional World Music."

Andi Goldman is a licensed psychotherapist specializing in holistic counseling and sound therapy. Andi and Jonathan have been married for over 20 years and have co-authored several books. These include *Chakra Frequencies: Tantra of Sound*, which received the 2006 Visionary Award for Best Alternative Health Book of the Year, and *The Humming Effect: Sound Healing for Health and Happiness*. Together Jonathan and Andi work to help heal and transform lives, conduct seminars, offer yoga retreats and several other programs, and also offer teacher training. Yogaville.org is their website where one can access a library of yoga classes including Hatha yoga, meditation, pranayama and more. The website healingsounds.com is a great resource for award winning sound healing music, reiki chants, Tibetan master chants and more.

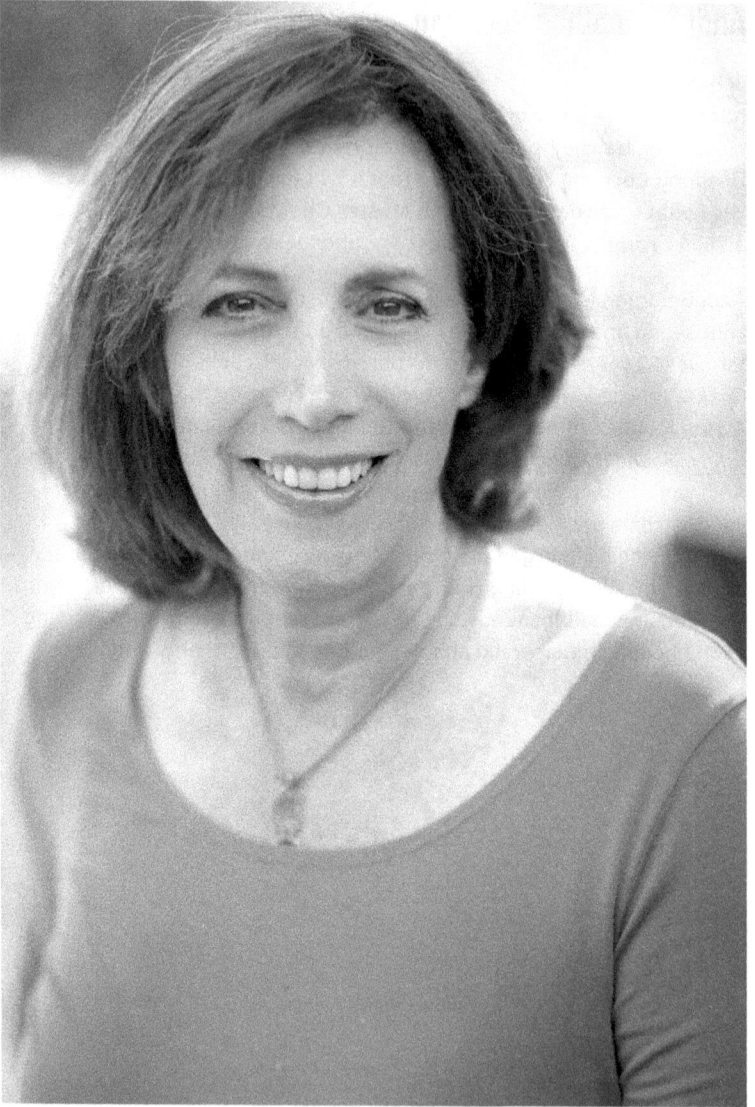

Beth Greer

Beth Greer

Beth Greer is Founder and CEO of The True Vitality Project. She is a healthy home transformer, detecting ways in which commonly used products and VOCs could be impacting health. She offers strategies, insights, and techniques you can use to transform your health and vitality. She is an award-winning journalist, stem cell activation advocate, and speaker on sustainable, natural living. Her journey of toxin-free living began after she was able to shrink a large chest tumor without surgery or drugs. She recommends use of a stem cell activating patch – a 100% natural way to stimulate natural healing within the body.

Beth is the author of *Super Natural Home: Improve Your Health, Home and Planet — One Room at a Time* endorsed by Deepak Chopra and Dr. Joseph Mercola. She can be found at supernaturalmom.com where she offers detox courses, health consulting, and in-home and remote home assessments. The website also carries a list of safe recommended products

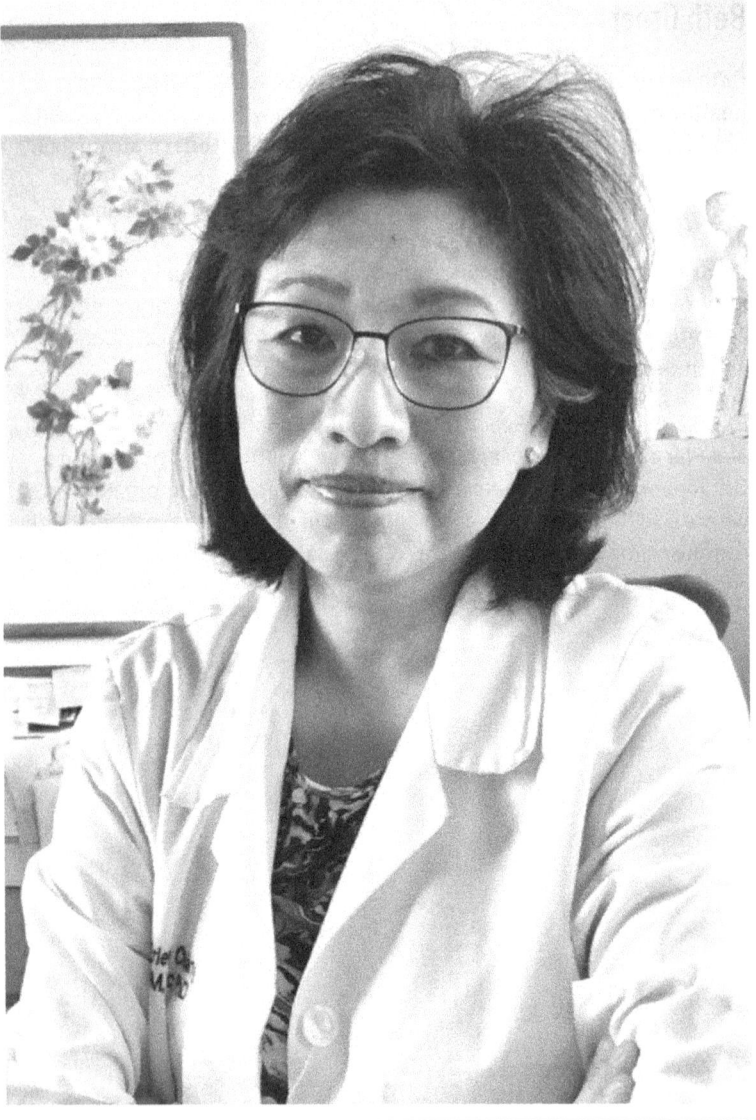

Dr. Erlene Chiang

Dr. Erlene Chiang

Dr. Erlene Chiang is a third generation traditional Chinese medicine practitioner. She has also served in the field of oncology as President, American Cancer Society, California Chinese Unit; Vice President, American Cancer Society; and Senior Administrative Director, California Chinese Unit. She's a faculty member of American College of Traditional Chinese Medicine at CIIS, and executive director of Wen Wu School of Martial Arts. She was also voted the Best Asian Herbalist by *East Bay Express*. She has published papers at *Journal of Acupuncture and Integrative Medicine*.

Her expertise in the areas of acupuncture, Qigong, and traditional herbal medicine means that she brings a unique holistic perspective to core cancer care, pain management, and other forms of healing. Dr. Chiang offers herbal medical treatments, acupuncture, and other therapies at the award winning Wen Wu School founded in 1972.

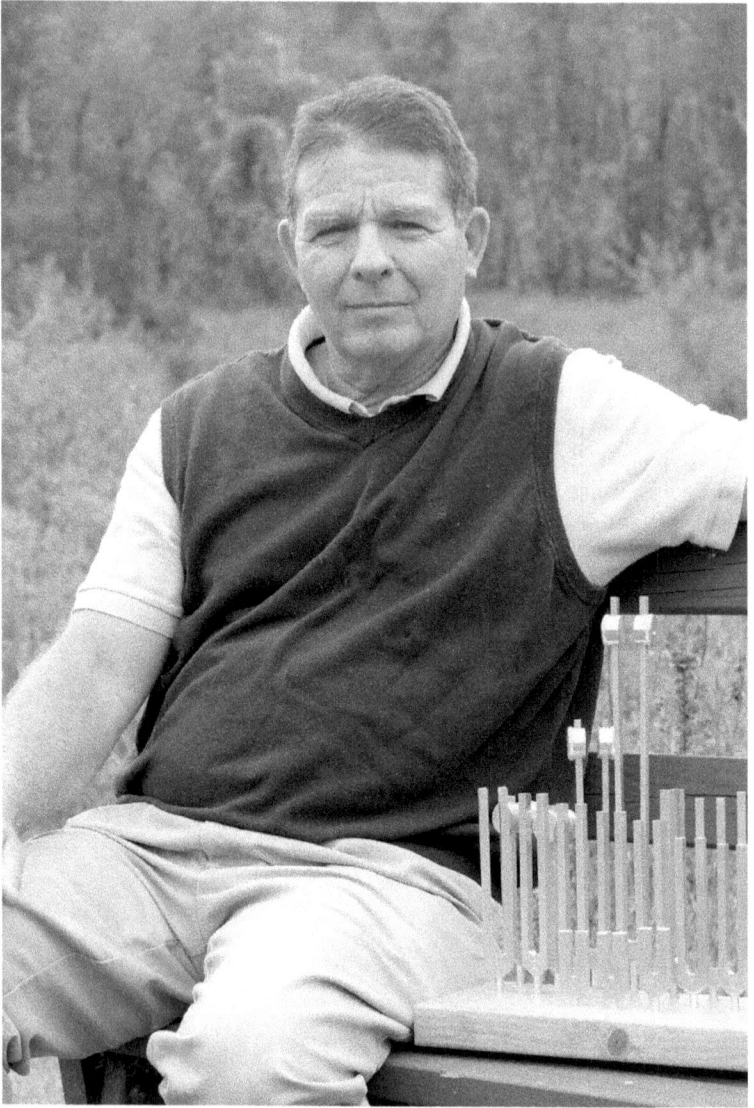

Dr. John Beaulieu

Dr. John Beaulieu

Dr. John Beaulieu is a sound healing innovator. He is a naturopathic physican and psychologist, as well as a composer, pianist, and philosopher. He is renowned for developing the BioSonic Repatterning™, which uses tuning forks for healing based on the sounds found in nature. Sound healing products such as the C & G tuning forks, crystal gem feet, color tuned glasses, and Dr. Beaulieu's books and research are available at biosonics.com. Dr. John Beaulieu's books include *Human Tuning*, *Sound Healing and Values Visualization*, *The Polarity Therapy Workbook*, and *Bellevue Memoirs*. Dr. Beaulieu's discography is free and available at biosonics1.bandcamp.com.

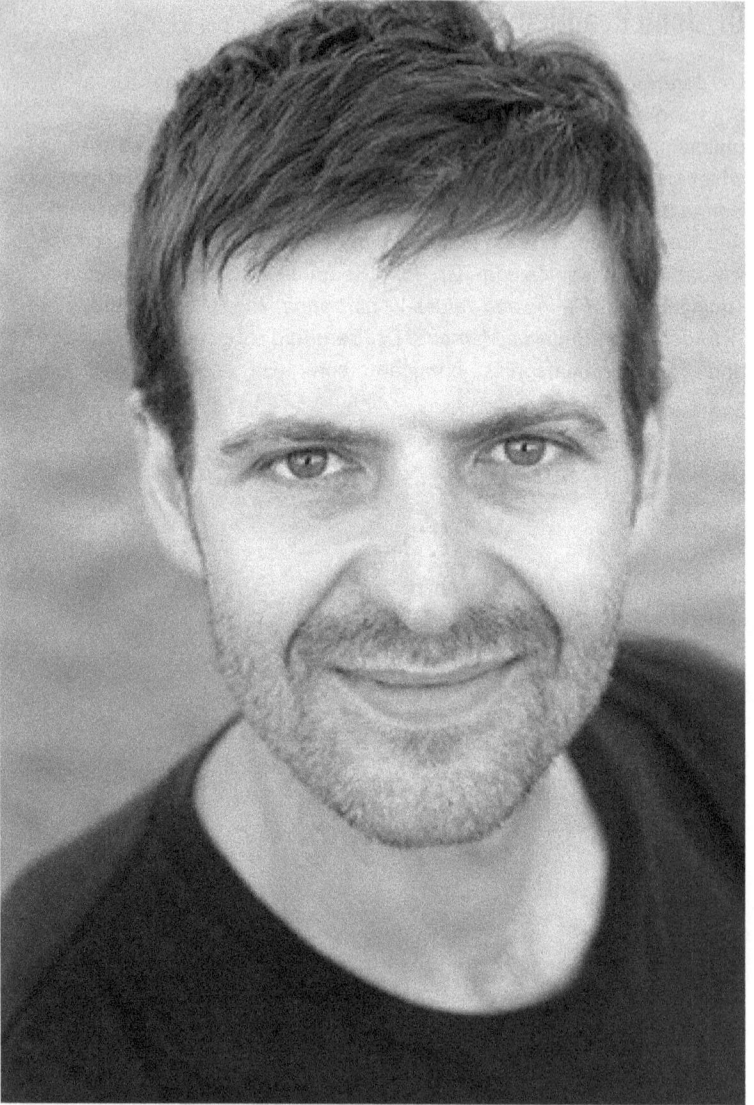

Jacob McGill

Jacob McGill

Having survived a very serious accident, coma, and months in hospital at age 17, Jacob McGill's journey of rehabilitation was also one of learning and discovery. He explored many different healing modalities, therapies, and nutritional approaches to overcome the pain and increase range of motion before deciding what really worked. He has since designed The Hundred Year Plan, a series of interventions designed to address chronic as well as acute pain emanating from injuries, repetitive stress, degenerative issues, and more. The program involves meditation, movement, important conversations with self, and breath-work. This is a comprehensive, online, movement-based rehabilitation system that helps avoid surgery and is seen to outperform physiotherapy. The program also includes breathing and postural correction techniques that directly address the underlying causes of pain.

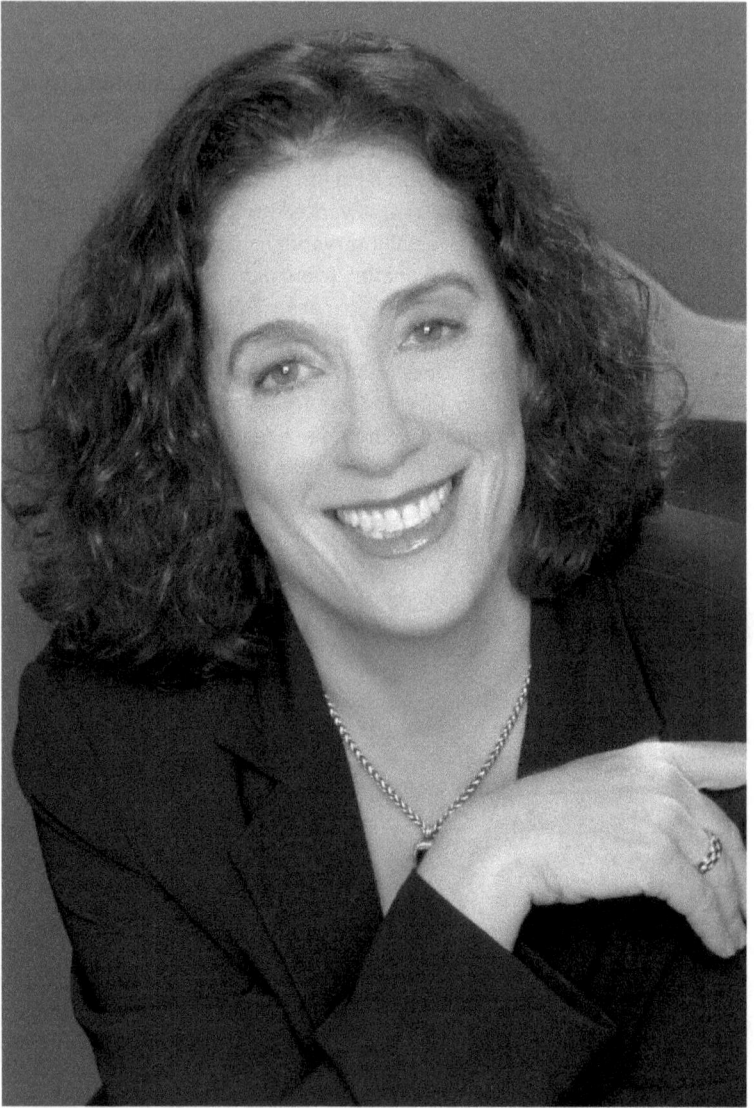

Anat Baniel

Anat Baniel

Anat Baniel is the best-selling author of *Move into Life* and the highly acclaimed *Kids Beyond Limits*, and founder of Anat Baniel Method® NeuroMovement® (ABMNM®) - a holistic approach to understanding learning, function, and acquisition of skills. Her work evolved from a background in dance, clinical psychology, and statistics, and from her close professional collaboration with Dr. Moshé Feldenkrais for over a decade. Anat and the hundreds of practitioners she has trained work with high performers such as athletes, musicians, and dancers, as well as those who suffered stroke, and people suffering from pain and limitations. She and her Method are world renowned for transforming the lives of children with special needs and their families.

Anat defined the *Nine Essentials* of NeuroMovement® that wake up the brain to rapid change, and offer practical, accessible methods to overcome pain, and increase flexibility, strength, creativity, and vitality by utilizing the power of neuroplasticity, coupled with the use of movement as a key driver of positive brain change. Her Method is supported by leading neuroscientists.

Anat believes that how we move is vital to the way we breathe, for our health, stamina, cognitive abilities, and even mood. It is possible to physically change our brain when we introduce change and variation in what we do and how we do it, she says. Moreover, conscious breathing can also help drive positive transformation.

Dr. Neil Sharp

Neil trained as a physician at Cambridge University and Edinburgh University Medical School. He subsequently left medicine to pursue a career in music as a professional opera singer. Discovering Anat Baniel and training in her work has allowed him to synthesize his passions and interests, and he now collaborates with her at her center in San Rafael California.

ENDNOTES

WHAT YOU DON'T KNOW CAN KILL YOU. KNOWLEDGE IS HEALTH
By Dr. Nathan S. Bryan

Source:

https://www.efsa.europa.eu/en/press/news/170615-0

https://onlinelibrary.wiley.com/doi/full/10.1002/fsn3.1

https://www.ncbi.nlm.nih.gov/pmc/articles/PMC3605573/

https://www.nobelprize.org/prizes/medicine/1998/press-release/

GETTING THE OXYGEN ADVANTAGE: BREATHE BETTER, FEEL BETTER
By Patrick McKeown

References:

1. https://podcasts.apple.com/es/podcast/185-life-lessons-from-a-brain-surgeon-with-dr-rahul-jandial/id1333552422?i=1000523107110

2. https://www.medicalnewstoday.com/articles/326831

3. https://time.com/4793331/instagram-social-media-mental-health/

4. http://www1.udel.edu/chem/white/C342/Bohr(1904).html

5. https://www.ncbi.nlm.nih.gov/pmc/articles/PMC5685417/

YOUR BREATH & HUMMING – CREATING THE VIBRATIONS THAT HEAL
By Andi & Jonathan Goldman

References:

1. https://www.physio-pedia.com/Therapeutic_Ultrasound

2. https://openarchive.ki.se/xmlui/bitstream/handle/10616/38896/thesis.pdf

3. https://www.ncbi.nlm.nih.gov/pmc/articles/PMC8117664/

4. https://www.amazon.com/Self-Healing-Techniques-Ranjie-Ph-D-Singh/dp/1896826008